I Got Sex at Comic-Con

—

A Fanboy Comic Book Geek's Move from Loser to Player

I0447516

David Banner

ACKNOWLEDGMENTS

Special thanks to Ben. S. and you know why.

A George OK'd the fact that I could live with having the upper-hand as I thought I was destined to do... but then a better George showed me how to lose the hand and be attractive to hot girls – *really* attractive to them!

And even with George, without Erik von Markovik my dating life would still be far more of a wasteland than the most amazing one it's become.

DEDICATION

Dedicated to Rose… of course.
We'll always have San Diego.

CONTENTS

I Got Sex at Comic-Con!

PREFACE
YOU'RE NOT GOING TO BELIEVE
WHAT I AM ABOUT TO TEACH YOU!

Each one of the events in this story is based on a true account. It reads like a story but it's full of facts my good friend.

Yeah, I got laid for the first time in my life at Comic-Con.

Normally that would be a miracle. But where this story really kicks butt is in *how* I got laid.

If you have as little success as I used to have with women, *I am about to give you the keys to the kingdom.*

Why do the jerks get all the women while we good guys stand around saying, "How does he do that?!" The answer is that the jerk understands women more than we do. It might come naturally or he may have been trained in how to do it. I am living proof that it's possible to be trained. In a few weeks, or sooner, you will be too.

I don't care how geeky you are. I don't care how fat, thin, bald, or hairy you are. I don't care if you swallow your tongue when a girl talks to you. Through my experience that culminated at Comic-Con, I am going to show you how to attract a female. I am going to tell you step-by-step how to get laid. You won't believe it… until you try it.

1
I WAS NOT JUST A LOSER BUT A SUPER-SIZED LOSER VIRGIN

It's a mixed blessing that my first name is David and not Bruce.

Most of the time I'm thrilled that my parents didn't name me Bruce. I avoided lame and illogical gay jokes my whole life just by not getting that first name. If you're named Bruce I'm not saying there's anything wrong with that name… But I am far less petty than many of my "friends" were whom I grew up with and I know what kind of life I would have had being named Bruce.

Worse than that, Bruce Banner is The Incredible Hulk's alter ego in the comics.

That green giant still haunted me however as some of you already have realized.

The drawback to being named David Banner is that more people seem to know that David Banner was the TV Hulk's alter ego than know that Bruce Banner was the Hulk's name in Marvel comics. Even though Bill Bixby played David

Banner as *The Incredible Hulk* way back in the late 1970s, people today still know the name and are always asking me, "What happens when *you* get angry?" and "Hey, don't go green on me man!" My response is usually something like, "Hmm, nobody has *ever* thought to say *that* to me before!"

The most amazing thing is they changed the character's name from Bruce to David precisely *because* the TV producers thought the name Bruce was gay-sounding! I heard that Stan Lee was pretty upset over that but I don't know if it's true. Either way, the whole thing's been a problem for me growing up.

And it was all made worse by the fact that I actually do love comic books, science fiction, fantasy (some fantasy), and everything that goes along with it. My own name sort of put a damper on my enjoyment of Hulk comics so I never really collected any of those. I missed a lot of good stories because of that. When the 2008 Hulk movie came out I had no idea that there was a lot of secondary stuff going on with the story. Like the fact that Samuel Sterns was a character introduced way back in the early 1960s.

Speaking of mixed blessings, it's also a mixed blessing that I've been a comic book collector since the age of seven.

From loving my comics at such a young age, my vocabulary and my reading skills exploded past all my classmates. The problem is that as my grades got better my success with girls decreased accordingly.

By the time I was 13 my hormones were raging and so was my acne. I was the typical idiot fanboy who immersed myself in my fantasy life without working on my social skills.

Man was I a dweeb. The guy in *Kick-Ass* was a stud and leading ladies man compared to me.

But all that changed.

I went to Comic-Con a virgin. I left Comic-Con a new man.

2
ALL THE HOT GIRLS WHO LIKED
ME LIVED ONLY IN MY DREAMS

I grew up knowing a lot of guys like me. We hung out together precisely because nobody cool would hang out with us. We were the fanboys, we had all the great sayings (like, *'Nuff said!* and *It's clobbering time!*), we were fairly intelligent as a group so our ability to talk sarcastically about the world around us was finely honed. We were like the kids in *Stand By Me* only with far less glitz and glamor than they had.

We had a lot in common when it came to girls too.

None of us had any.

None of us had a girlfriend and none of us had a date – if you don't count my cousin Tina who went to an 8th grade science fair with George because he rode with her and her Mom, my Aunt, who was volunteering to help the school during the fair. George came home really liking Tina. Tina went home really disgusted with George because he kept telling her how much she looked like Sue Richards.

George, whose full name is George Pilkington, was always pudgy. He wasn't obese but his jeans always rolled down over the top of his belt because as soon as his Mom got him new jeans he would grow another size in the belly. When he stopped growing at "husky" she stopped buying him jeans. So the roll was always there.

And if I hated the name David Banner, George truly seethed at the name George. Because for a guy like him it *is* a dorky name.

For a guy like George Clooney, George is not a dorky name. For a guy like George Pilkington, George is a dorky name. My buddy George Pilkington *defined* dork just by his presence.

Yes, I Still Find it Hard to Believe

I'll give you a sneak preview of how this book ends.

George, as in George Pilkington, as in my dork friend for the last 16 years, was the reason why I got laid at Comic-Con. I got laid because he taught me exactly how to get laid.

But it only works with beautifully stunning women. So if you're not into 9's and 10s then look elsewhere. For example, these tactics don't work on the majority of chicks who frequent comic book conventions. But at the giant Comic-Con in San Diego, the girls who are 10's are actually plentiful there. Many are working the show but many are also attending.

George's Metamorphosis

George turned from, well, from *George* to a woman-magnet in one summer. Last summer George went to his brother's in Maine and stayed for two months. His older brother Rick was always cool. I still remember Rick living at home before he grew up and went to Maine on a new job he got. He was nice to all of us in spite of how backwards we all were. Rick seemed happy to see us and always helped us when we needed help, like when he built a skate ramp for us.

And Rick always had the babes. If he wasn't going out on a date he was coming home from one.

Rick was the exact, twin, mirror-image of George. No, not George his brother. George Clooney.

Only Rick didn't *look* like Clooney. Rick wasn't all that handsome. He wore some weird stuff like big and gaudy rings and purple vests and things like that. His hair was never cut all that well. His voice was not as suave as Clooney's. And yet, Rick always had this charming appeal that I couldn't define really. At least I couldn't back then. I now know what was going on. I understand his attraction and I now know how to fake the same attraction. You will too.

But back then, I knew I just liked him and everybody else did to.

Especially the ladies.

And to this day it amazes me that I never questioned why they liked Rick. If I had studied the situation a little I may have gotten laid far sooner. But those aren't the kinds of things one thinks about studying. It took George to learn what Rick was doing to get laid and then to pass along all the secrets to me.

George Comes Through – Oh Man Did He!

As I said, George was the reason I got laid at Comic-Con. George the dorky but faithful friend. George who went to Maine and came home a changed man. Maine changed George as much as Comic-Con changed me. The coolest thing about George is that he is a true friend. He knew I was as much of a loser as he was. The pre-Maine George that is.

So he taught me the things that Rick taught him in Maine.

Let me tell you clearly – the things George taught me would be worth fortunes to some Kings. Wealthy men would trade countless stacks of gold to know what George learned last summer from Rick. You're lucky. You only paid a little for my book. I should have charged more money for it.

Forget the Lies

I always heard this phrase: "The girls I like *never* want anything to do with me. The ones that like me are horrible."

What a lie.

I never understood why guys would say that and gripe about it. I heard guys say it, no guy from my immediate circle, but others right outside our circle whom we interacted with a lot. You know, the non-jocks, the guys who were nice, didn't have tremendous success with girls, but did well in school, stayed under the radar, and were sort of our connection to the upper-tiered people. Through this next level on the school hierarchy, we could learn about people who would never have anything to do with my immediate group of friends.

I especially remember a guy named Eddie Tucker. He was in that next-up strata of people. He never liked comics or movies or things like those but we got along okay. One afternoon, we were talking about how hard it is to talk to girls and he said the old, "Girls I like *never* want me. Girls who do want me, like Harriett Laramie, are ugly."

I thought, "Why are you bitching Eddie? If a girl likes you even if she is ugly or whatever you based the term 'horrible' on, well at least she's a girl! At least she likes you! At least you have someone to call at night! At least you have a warm body to dance with at the prom!"

But I didn't say it to him. Eddie probably would have still been my friend but I as always careful. I could say anything to George and the others in my group and they'd still like me but I never risked Eddie's friendship. He was a step above my usual buddy and I had to keep him in hopes of someday moving up to that next strata.

Why didn't guys like Eddie just go ahead and hang out with the girls who liked them? Harriett, for example, was *not* ugly. She was sort of plain and she was sort of whiny but she was a *she!* Harriett Laramie was actually a pretty good friend of mine at school. She never showed any interest in me other than as a friend and I never had any interest in her really but we got along and hung out some. Harriett had sort of a funny lip. It wasn't anything that needed surgery but it was just sort of a misshapen mouth and Harriett wasn't all that nice to be around except to me. And Eddie Tucker. She had such a crush on him for about 2 years. She always wanted me to talk to Eddie about her. They knew each other but she kept thinking I could somehow get him to like her if I talked her up enough to him.

I could say she was crazy but I'd probably do the same thing. If I knew a girl well who knew another girl I really liked, I'd almost certainly try to get my friend to tell the babe something to generate an interest in me since I didn't have any guts to try.

I told you I was a loser.

But the bottom line is that Eddie refused to like Harriett back. She just wasn't quite in his league. And what he didn't realize was that his league was about a hair above *my league* and my league had as much a chance at getting a cool girl as we had at making the varsity football team.

But let me get back to the lie of the day growing up: "The girls I like *never* want anything to do with me. The ones that like me are horrible."

For guys like me and George, even the horrible ones didn't want us. We could lust after the 9's and 10's. We could fantasize about the 7's and 8's. We could think about asking out the 4's, 5's, and 6's even though we never did. And the reality was that the 1's, 2's, and 3's had more self-worth than to be interested in the geeks who traded each other comics in elementary school, game cards in middle school, and sci-fi movies in high school.

The 1's through the 5's used *us* to get the guys on the next-level up. The Harriett's used us to try to get the Eddies

I would have appreciated a Harriett. I thought. What did I know? Any port in the storm.

But all the girls who liked me, even the ones I'd lower my standards for, only liked me in my dreams. As far as I know there was never a girl, good or bad, who liked me.

What a loser I was.

3
GIRLS AND GEEKS GO TOGETHER
LIKE CLARK KENT AND KRYPTONITE

It's not a big secret. Fanboys just don't get the women.

What do we like that *they* like? Nothing.

I'd often look around my room and see posters and comics and game cards and movies and think this: "Someday, I will meet a cool girl who not only is going to like all this but she will be into it as much as she is into me!"

Once in a while partial reality would set in. Through a far-off lens, I learned a lot about girls all around me. I'd listen to them as I passed them in the halls with my eyes down. I'd watch them arrive to class talking about their night, the one before or the next one coming up. I'd read a lot of the blogs of the cool girls at school (that was fairly painful for me because it just confirmed how little chance I had with any of them).

The reality came in waves every couple of months when I took an inventory of all I knew about all the girls in my school. And *not one of them was into comics, game cards, sci-fi, Xbox, or anything else that my room reeked of.*

And I'd just be sad. All the time and money I invested in all that stuff not only didn't get me closer to the only thing I really wanted, companionship, but it did the opposite. The more I was into all the things I loved, the less I'd be into girls who could love me.

Changing Wouldn't Have Mattered

I considered throwing away *everything* and becoming normal. You know, liking books that didn't have a protagonist who was either fanged, caped, or from another planet. Well I wouldn't have thrown them away. I would have sold it all on eBay. I suspect I'd be about $15,000 wealthier if I'd done that.

Looking back, knowing then what I know now, it turns out that doing away with all that stuff wouldn't have helped on the chick front. I would not have been different. I'd still be just a geeky guy who no longer owned a bunch of geeky stuff. I am glad I kept it because it got my mind off how bad off I was in the relationship department.

Other than the girls, I was fairly happy. My mom was sort of cool for a divorced mom in a medium-sized Arizona town who worked a lot. She trusted me to be alone while she was working which was fine by me. At the same time, I was such a loser why would she have anything to worry about? It's not like I would be going to all the parties in town, throwing back brewskies and shots with the jocks, and getting all the party skirts pregnant.

I liked hanging out with George and Enzo and Frank, my three buddies, my companions-in-geek. I learned to appreciate the stories of the comics as the entire comic industry matured, especially when I started reading back issues from the 1990s when series such as *The Watchmen* and much of Frank Miller's work propelled the stories and art forward about 100 light years over the more traditional fare of the 1960s through the late 1980s.

The stories and all that goes with liking them, including the game cards, science-fiction and fantasy books and movies, electronic games, and the like got me through week after week of what otherwise could have been a severe funk and depression. Yes, looking back now I would *not* have been any better off in the girl department if I'd not had all that stuff.

I certainly wouldn't have gone to Comic-Con and gotten laid.

4
THE CHANGE YOU
MAKE TO GET LAID

I know you're tired of hearing me rant on and on about my B.S. (*Before Sex*) life.

Nevertheless, if you are relating to anything I'm telling you about my B.S. life then all of this serves its purpose. I want you to know that I was in the gutter looking up just to see the slime in the gutter when it came to women. I want you to know that I had as much chance of getting laid at Comic-Con as you probably do right now.

Let's face it; you're reading some geek's account of how he popped his cherry instead of getting your own popped.

But you're going to pop yours if you keep reading. You are going to be stunned. You are going to be shocked when you see how to do it. And it works. For guys like me. Yes, for guys just like you.

It turns out that all the comic book stuff was doing nothing to hurt me getting a girl. It wasn't helping but it was not my crutch or excuse. *I* was the excuse. I was stopping myself.

So are you.

And all those reasons going through your head *right now* – the reasons that what I'm about to teach you won't work for you are nothing but vaporware. The things I'm about to teach you *will work for you.*

If you clam up and can't talk to women, it won't matter.

If you *can* talk to women but say nothing but stupid things, it won't matter.

If you are fat, bald, thin, hairy, short, or anything else, it won't matter.

Think of every excuse in the book why you fail on the skirt front and put it in the following blank space: If you _____, it won't matter.

I wouldn't have believed it either. And you've already bought this book, you might as well finish it right? You might as well get laid because you've invested the time reading so far.

My Dream Girl

I always thought I could use my love of comics to get girls. Yeah, that is about as insane as Michael Moore going on a diet but I believed it. I thought my passion was so strong that it would carry over. The sci-fi universe I enjoyed would be fodder to show women that yes, they were geeky *but* that comics were not comic books but *graphic novels.*

One problem with that theory is I never could get past having to start a conversation with a good-looking female. In other words, I couldn't explain that my love of Marvel comics wasn't childish because I couldn't talk to a girl in the first place.

How does one go up to Elizabeth Sanders in her cheerleader uniform and start talking to her?

The next problem is that if I could find a way to start a conversation – perhaps if she dropped a book and I picked it up and talked to her – segueing to the realm of comics would be an impossible task. It's not as though she'd thank me for the book and I'd be all debonair and reply, "No thanks is necessary, I'm always happy to help. Oh, and speaking of Happy, do you think Happy Hogan is ever going to hook up with Pepper Potts or do you think Iron Man would get too jealous?"

A couple of years ago I realized that the comics were *not* going to help with women in any way, shape, or form. If I marginalized the comics I might be able to get away with keeping that as my hobby as long as the girl liked me for my other qualities. But I had no qualities a girl would like.

"Be Yourself, You'll Find a Nice Girl!"

This is the king of the king of all lies.

"Be yourself!"

I had been being myself ever since I reached puberty. Myself was someone who had no idea how to approach a girl and have no idea what to say once I did. Myself was someone with no attribute that would attract a girl.

If you think the best way of you getting laid is to "be yourself," how has that been working out for you?

The second-biggest king of lies is: "You'll find a nice girl. Girls want boys they can trust, boys they can talk to, boys who aren't jerks."

Now that the scales have fallen from my eyes I realize the previous statement isn't necessarily false. Its problem is that nice boys and trust-worthy boys are not attractive to girls. We might be the guys they fantasize about settling down with but we are *not* the guys they fantasize about settling down with *tonight*.

Nice guys finish last and if you think that is cliché, let me ask again: How has being yourself and being nice been working out for you so far?

Take everything you know about getting laid right now. Throw it in the trash.

Are You This Guy?

Since George gave me the keys to the kingdom and showed me exactly how to get girls, and I am talking about going from 0 to 100 MPH with 9's and 10's, I have noticed a trend among "nice guys."

It's not a universal trend among guys like me but it's fairly common. I can now spot a "nice guy," meaning a guy who never has dates on Friday nights. He almost always has these characteristics:

- Wears polo shirts and often nice T-shirts *always tucked in*.

- Has his hair combed and every hair in place.

- Walks down the hall looking a little timid but always wearing a friendly face.

- Is always clean and neat.

- Often has high intelligence.

- Never smiles but never grimaces. He is neutral.

- He might smile *if* a girl happens to look at him (but has no idea what to say).

- If a girl *does* talk to him, his grammar is perfect and he is about as polite as Alfred the Butler.

I also now notice common characteristics of guys who always have dates on Friday nights.

They almost always:

- Wear more grungy clothes; maybe they are clean clothes but often not tucked in.

- Walks down the halls, often talking louder than other guys, and not paying too much attention to the women looking at them.

- He strikes up conversations with his buddies as he passes them.

- He glances at the women, smiling before and after seeing them, but rarely says more than "Hey" to them as he moves.

The star jocks always have these characteristics but jocks aren't the only guys with dates on Friday nights. There are lots of non-jocks without much going for them who have women all the time. These were always the guys that stunned me. I understood that girls would love the muscles on the jocks but other guys didn't have *anything* on me physically. And they weren't as well-groomed as me!

Yet they had girls. These non-jocks who didn't have the looks. All my politeness and shirt-tucking in the world did nothing to get me a girl.

I now understand it all. You will too. I understand that there was not magic in the non-jocks who got the girls. Yeah, they had all the funny characteristics I list above, ones that any mother would tell you are the worst characteristics compared to nice guys like me.

And it turns out that they didn't care about their grooming less than I did. It turns out they didn't disrespect women more than I did. The theme turns out to be this: lo and behold, as they get more and more girls those bad characteristics are reinforced by the girls! As the jocks and non-jocks got dates and had a little early success with girls if they began tucking in their shirts and showing a lot of interest in the females then they would *stop* getting as many girls. Just through an unconscious trial and error, they learned what to do and how to behave to get the skirts.

This Isn't About Being a Jerk

The phrase "Nice guys finish last" is true about guys like me when it comes to girls. But one can't be a jerk to women and all of a sudden they get laid.

There is something in-between and it's a magical place indeed. A place that you can learn easily. There is a place you can get to fast, just by learning a few basics, memorizing a few conversation threads, where you can strike the balance of not being so nice you turn off a girl and not being so rude you turn off a girl.

I thought there were only two states: polite and rude.

There is a third state: She wants you and has no idea why.

This is the state those guys are in who sort of smile as they glance to then away at women but greet and high-five their buddies as they walk down the hall. And it's a state you will master quickly. Because at first it will be rote to you just as it is to me. But your success with women will quickly reinforce your characteristics so you naturally enter that state and become the guy you never thought you'd become: A geek who gets laid.

If you play it right and practice, you can even keep your comics! They won't care!

I find, however, that I desire the comics less and the girls more as I get more and more girls.

Knowledge is All You Lack

You only lack knowledge.

You don't need a better haircut. Probably you need to fiddle with your hair less.

You don't need a new wardrobe. Probably you need to take your wardrobe less seriously than you already do. Untuck, that shirt soldier!

You don't need a personality makeover. You just need to memorize a surprisingly few phrases and lines.

You don't need to work out in the gym. I have started working out but only so I can have a little more *oomph* in bed; I certainly don't work out to *get* girls. That would be *way* too much work.

You only lack knowledge.

Hygiene is Vital

Men, I just have to tell it to you straight. You've gotta be clean.

You can be somewhat scruffy looking in clothing and hair and all of that. But you need to be clean. Unless you just threw the homecoming varsity game's winning touchdown and ran off the field to cheers, don't have B.O.

Take a shower every day, keep your breath fresh, and make sure your clothes which might be slightly unkept are still clean.

If you are overweight, be honest with yourself when it comes to odors. If you aren't overweight, be honest with your odors!

The jock's jock won't get a date if he stinks.

Other than that, you don't need to do much in the grooming department except worry far less about grooming than you used to if you never left the house with your ironed Polo shirt tucked into your pants.

5
GEORGE DROPS THE BOMBSHELL

Here is the starting point of how I went from loser B.S. life to getting laid at Comic-Con in less than 6 months. And you can move from Before Sex faster than I did. I'm a better teacher than George.

George got home from his cool brother Nick's house in Maine. I thought he'd be banging on my door within minutes of his parents picking him up from the airport. We'd discussed a lot of fanboy news about some new graphic novels and movie deals through emails while he was gone and some of the news was fairly juicy, especially the rumors that surrounded the next *Avengers* movie that actually looked as though it would not only get made but be pretty good.

But I had to call George the day after he got home. And all was okay, he wasn't *extremely* different. But somewhat he was. Something was off. I didn't get the cold shoulder; he was nice to me as always and he talked over some recent news. We discussed driving together to Comic-Con the following July. We discussed being Seniors at school. We discussed all the things we'd normally discuss.

I would turn 18 in just 60 days because I was a little older than most in my class and George wasn't too far behind me. We discussed that this was the year before college and we had no idea whether we'd go or sit out a year or two first.

But George just didn't have the energy he had before he went to Nick's. He seemed… a little more mature than he should have been.

This was the start of 2 or 3 months of George and I drifting apart.

I Meet my Best Friend Again for the First Time in December

With school starting and classes being harder than ever (geeks almost always ended up in the advanced placement classes), George and I saw less of each other and I didn't think a lot about it. I thought George was a little aloof but it wasn't all his fault. Our lunch schedules didn't match for the first time and I had a part-time job after school at an Optician's place grinding eye glass lens. ("I jumped into the grinder once and made a spectacle out of myself!" I'd be in the back of the shop grinding out the lenses each day on this somewhat computerized but gritty grinder and I'd think of all sorts of zingers related to my job. "…and made a spectacle of myself!" Oh I had a million such lines! But I had no girl.)

At Thanksgiving Break my Mom and I went to my grandparents in New Mexico. It was kind of cool because they live in the same area where they were filming *Breaking Bad* and I saw some of the filming once when we visited in February. I saw a lot of places that were shown as background in the show.

But my point here is that I didn't see George at Thanksgiving when we'd normally spend 24/7 with each other. And by then, we saw and spoke very little. It was sort of weird but other stuff filled my life and I didn't think too much about it.

Until Christmas Break. We had two weeks and the first three days I spent trying to connect with George. In those three days he was home only one time when I called and said he would have to call me back. Six days later, well into the second week of break, he called in the morning and simply said, "I need to see you."

Okay. Er, ... okay. "Dude," I said in my usual brilliance, "you didn't turn gay on me did you? You *need* to see me?"

He quipped back, fairly short-tempered, and said, "I need to see you." He used his serious voice. Something was wrong. The entire semester we just finished came flashing through my mind and I realized in four months I had lost my best friend and didn't even realize it.

I said, "Sure George. Come on over."

"No. Can you be at Carlos's tonight at 6:30?"

Carlos's Pies was a local pizza place we liked a lot. The pizza wasn't great but it was cheap. And they had fairly good games that they actually changed out every few months for variety. And they had WiFi so we could go online. And they had far more take-out business than dine-in so we could sit there for 3 or 4 hours on a night like that (Tuesday) and nobody cared.

I agreed to meet George at Carlos's place.

We always split a large pie and I can always eat my half with ease and George always eats his and wants more.

I went to Carlos curious about George but also extremely hungry. I didn't eat much for lunch because I hadn't been to Carlos's Pies since the previous Spring when George and I hung out there putting the finishing touches on a joint lab project for Biology. We ate at Carlos's every night for eight days straight working on that project's big report. It had been so long, my taste buds watered all day thinking about the pizza. I decided that it had been so long, if I ate my half and was in the least bit hungry, I'd order a second pizza.

We met and ordered our usual Large Canadian Bacon with extra cheese. George had changed in one obvious way. He was wearing some of his brother Nick's big, gaudy rings and a watch and a necklace! A necklace, George! But what could I say? Nothing was off limits when it came to giving George a hard time but those were Nick's things and I knew he loved his brother Nick more than any of us and we all loved Nick. So I didn't say much about the jewelry but I thought it was a little silly on George. It sure stood out on him, not only because George is pudgy but shorter than Nick so anything that accented any part of him like rings and watches and necklaces just looked more silly.

Anyway, we sat down and the pizza came in a few minutes. Carlos was as fast as I was hungry. Before George had his pulled away from the pan, I had eaten an entire slice. Man that was a good slice.

As I was gobbling down the slice, I said, "George, man, why don't I ever see you? I know we don't have classes together but we never had to work so hard to get together before now!"

George said something that was The Most Unbelievable Thing I had ever heard him say in his life. And George always said crazy things that weren't true.

As his told me that sentence, The Most Unbelievable Thing I had ever heard George say, I instantly knew George was not exaggerating this time. Something was clear and that something was that George was stating simple truth.

I swallowed the last of that first piece of pizza I had gobbled in the seconds before George said that. And I did not eat another bite… the rest of the evening.

We stayed five and a half hours, leaving only because Carlos came over and said, "Guys I've got to close for the night."

George's Transformation

Again, my question as I gobbled my first and last slice of pizza was this: "George, man, why don't I ever see you? I know we don't have classes together but we never had to work so hard to get together before now!"

George replied: "I've been dating way too much to hang out with you. I'm sorry, I need to stop going out with so many skirts so we can spend more time together."

6
GEORGE GOT THE TORCH, THEN PASSED IT TO ME

I was about to begin my journey that you are now about to begin.

Nick Comes Through for George...

It turns out George got to Nick's place and sort of had a break-down. George didn't talk too much about that but he didn't seem embarrassed by it. There was just no reason to go into all the details with me.

George got to Nick's place and after a couple of days Nick asked his little brother about the dating world back here in Real Life, USA. George asked, "How would I know Nick?" and Nick replied with something like, "George, are you crazy? The women back home are crazy for guys. You should be cleaning up better than I ever did and I did just fine!"

At that point, it seems George just broke down balling.

I'm not giving George a hard time over this. I probably would have broken down too if I had a stud brother who got women easier than The Joker gets laughs. Over the course of that day, George taught Nick what it's like being Guys Like Us.

Nick had no idea. He just figured George had followed in his footsteps back home, taking up the slack, entertaining the ladies, and being happy as can be. Nick spent the next two months showing George how to get girls.

...and George Comes Through for Me

George spent the next 5 days of our break teaching me the basics. And the next month expanding on the basics. And he took me for the next 3 months out a couple of times a week giving me "field training."

In the time between leaving Nick's house with a mind full of newfound knowledge and a mouth full of memories of girl saliva he tasted in Maine, George honed the skills his brother told him about when he got back home. By "pizza night" with me, he was like a highly-skilled surgeon.

And he was ready to show me what he knew.

7
A SUB-CULTURE YOU
NEVER KNEW EXISTED

Just as George honed his knowledge and skills, honestly I surpassed George in next few months. I had a drive to research more at first and that gave me a time advantage over George who did more field work sooner. George began having extreme girl success in Maine with his brother but he got *really* good once he got back here to Arizona in an environment he was familiar with.

Once he told me about the whole skill set, I took it to new levels of knowledge.

I know that Nick did the right thing getting George out to clubs fast to get his hesitation killed before it got so bad that George would let it overcome him. I learn more by books than through experiential learning and I did a little more online and book learning before doing much in the field. It was probably harder for me when I first went out, but George was there to help some. But I think I progressed faster than George.

I know that 3 times I could have gotten laid in the months before Comic-Con. And if you had told me 6 months before that that I would be saying the previous sentence, I would ask what it is you've been smoking.

My problem is that I now had the ability but not the place! I lived with Mom and the girls my age did too. I should maybe have gone after slightly older women who had their own place but there is something *so satisfying* as getting dates with girls who did not know you existed for the entire decade you'd been sitting next to them in class. There was something incredibly alluring to getting dates with the 9's and 10's, the girls that were so good I never fantasized about *them* because fantasy has to have *some* basis in reality! My fantasies were with the 7's and 8's.

But I never got to third base with 7's and 8's after George taught me what Nick taught him. I never did make out with 7's and 8's because there were far too many 9's and 10's to work through.

And by Comic-Con, the 9's and 10's were easy for me to get. The difference in San Diego is that Comic-Con gave me a *place* to do something about it.

7's and 8's? 9's and 10's? Sexist Pig?

I'm writing this man-to-man.

Well, actually I'm writing this man-to-geek loser.

And I can say geek loser because I was far more of one than you could ever be.

Fortunately, the bridge from geek loser-to-man is far shorter than you ever thought possible.

Still. I'm writing this assuming other guys are reading it. If your sensibilities are damaged by me objectifying women by referring to them on a relative scale such as 8's and 10's then you need to close this book now and go back to *X-Men Unlimited*.

First of all there is an entire language surrounding the skills I'm going to teach you here. And this language allows us to short-cut the training. And being able to say things such as:

"This works on the 10's but not on the 7's"

is far clearer and faster for you to grasp than if I said:

"This works on beautiful girls, or the ones extremely confident in themselves, who dress to the hilt and who are looking for the top-tiered men. Surprisingly, the skills don't work as well on the girls who are not so… well, so GREAT and snobby – you know, the ones that actually say 'Hi' to you in class when they sit in front of you even if you never stand a chance of dating anyone of their caliber. The most beautiful and confident girls always seem to have an entourage around them and this works because of the group dynamics they bring to the social situation. A girl who is not quite as pretty and who is less confident will not react the same way because their interactions with other guys are far different and you must handle them a lot differently. The bottom line is that it's far easier to get a date with a beautiful, confident, socially-adept female than one who is more average."

Come on! Talking like, "This works on the 10's but not on the 7's" means we can get you trained faster so put away your little-boy fantasies about being a prince who only speaks about ladies and never about 10's.

I'm going to call them *10's* and I'm going to call them *4's* and I'm going to call them *skirts* and I'm going to use the outdated term *chicks* and I'm going to use language that was developed for this whole skill set and you can either man-up and learn it or – if learning this new way of talking is too foreign to you then go back to your Klingon Dictionary and keep practicing that. You won't ever have a date but you will get the nuances of the next *Star Trek* novel you read this coming cold, lonely Friday night.

This Sub-Culture

As I said there is an entire sub-culture out there that you didn't know existed. I am now a part of what I had no clue about a year ago. If every guy knew about this, perhaps it would be less effective. But the truth is, 99% of guys don't know about any of it and the 1% that do are mostly bad at it. They short-circuit so much of it that they do have more success than other men but they would have so much more if they just put a little effort into honing and perfecting the skills.

This sub-culture has been around for centuries but really didn't become standardized and honed and written about in textbook-like form until the late 1990s and early 2000s. This is the sub-culture called *The Pick-Up Artist*, or the *PUA*.

Perhaps hearing the term Pick-Up Artist makes you think of the old Dean Martin movies with the men holding martinis and sweet-talking the sultry platinum blondes. Maybe you think of AMC's *Mad Men* and think, that's way too suave to work in today's world. You are correct. The PUA sub-culture promotes skills that work almost flawlessly in today's world with today's girls. Today's PUA sub-culture is far different from the 1950s martini-driven man/woman interaction. But the results are the same. You get the chicks. And you get the dynamite ones, not the 5's.

The modern PUA sub-culture is not unlike the comic book/fanboy sub-culture. The big difference is the world doesn't know much about the PUA subculture. The world does know that we comic book geeks exist. Oh, and another difference is one sub-culture has zero girls and one is flooded with girls, all of whom are 9's and 10's.

It turns out there are people who travel the world giving training seminars for loser guys like you and (formerly) me. They charge thousands of dollars teaching them what I'm going to show you here. There are books out there, some of which I am going to suggest you get after you read this one. There are movies and TV shows too. Tons of web sites exist, some good and most bad.

But in spite of the plethora of materials out there, many of which stray way too far from the basics, *hardly anybody knows it all exists*! Statistically, the PUA sub-culture doesn't exist. This is good for you. There is an entire set of 9's and 10's all around you who have to put up daily with idiot guys attempting to get dates with them using all the same techniques that fail every time they're tried.

Watch from afar the 9's and 10's the next time you're in a large social setting like a club. Watch those women you would have never thought about talking to and see how obvious it is, now that you know what to look for, that they are sick and tired of being hit on the same way by the same idiots. Often good-looking idiots, but idiots nonetheless.

The field is ripe for you to step in and approach them the way *they want to be approached.*

In other words, you are going to learn not only how to approach a 9 or 10 but how a 9 or 10 wants to be approached but rarely or never is.

8
YOUR TRAINING BEGINS

I am going to fast forward from this point on.

You need less back-and-forth conversation between George and me. Still, I am going to include various conversational sections that George told me that night and over time and various questions I had for him along the way. But I'm switching now to more of a textbook approach. This writing just went from mostly sounding like a story to mostly being a non-fiction, step-by-step, how-to guide for getting dates with 9's and 10's.

You need no more gritty details of my boring life to this point. You are now ready for this book's Act 2, the act that benefits you the most.

George Taught Great Things But He Didn't Teach Well

At Carlos's, George was all over the map when he began telling me how to get the women. He raised far more questions than answers. Part of the problem was that he was taught over two months by Rick and Rick wasn't a good teacher either. But Rick's excuse is that much of the PUA came naturally to him. He was getting women and neither he nor others really knew why. It was just he was a natural leader and everybody liked Rick. The opposite of George and me.

George taught all this to me ass-backwards because he will always be George and he will always be a pudgy, nerdy guy who can't put two thoughts together sequentially.

The only difference between the B.S. George and the P.S. George is that now he is a pudgy, nerdy guy who gets laid all the time. Before Sex George no longer exists.

But my point for you is this: I have worked on the rest of this book for a long time. I originally wrote it the way George taught all this to me and *none of it made any sense*. It dawned on me after about the 45th re-write why it wasn't working. I went through problems of understanding and made a lot of mistakes that I would not have gone through had George just taught everything to me in a logical, ordered, systematic way.

But George is anything but logical, ordered, and systematic.

He taught me for example how to escalate the physical touching with a woman – no, not foreplay, just casual touching which is so vital to moving forward and not getting stuck in the "let's just be friends" stage. Many guys like me who do get the guts to talk to girls and get to know them almost always fall into the dreaded "let's just be friends" stage. This is because they are so nice to the girl that they never close the attraction switch in her mind. They would never touch a woman, even just a casual arm touch because they want her to know they respect her.

They never touch her when getting to know her and therefore they never get to touch her afterwards either.

So I scrubbed all I'd written for the rest of this book and came back here to re-work everything he taught me. I *am* a logical, ordered, systematic guy. I am going to give you the works, exactly what to learn, exactly what to say, and exactly how to move as you say it.

You Are About to Learn How to Get a Girl

You are going to learn how to get a girl for a date if that's all you want.

You are going to learn how to get a girl for sex if that's all you want.

You are going to learn how to get a girlfriend if that's what you want.

You are going to learn how to get a future wife if that's what you want.

9

GROUP DYNAMICS,
AN INTRODUCTION

Let's begin with a quiz. Suppose strikingly sexy Sally
Simpson is the girl you decide you want. Whatever you
define "want" as, whether it's sex, a date, marriage, or all of
the above, works for this quiz.

Which scenario is easiest to get a date with strikingly sexy
Sally Simpson?

- *Scenario One*: Sally is sitting in a local coffee shop at 3:00
  in the afternoon with only four other customers in the
  place. She's sitting alone, not all the way in the back,
  but at a table sipping her cappuccino, looking through a
  magazine. (You have two classes together with Sally,
  but she's a 10 and wouldn't know that.) The day is
  bright, the weather is perfect, people are all happy

inside. You order your coffee and walk by her. As you do, Sally looks up at you.

- *Scenario Two*: Sally is clubbing with her three friends, all of whom are 9.5's (Sally's a 10 of course). The noise level is at atmospheric levels, the four of them are facing each other in a circle not paying much attention to all the bodies and noise around them, and in order for you to get close enough to yell your words so Sally can hear you, you must squeeze through a line of jocks who can crush you with their pinkies.

Obviously the answer is Scenario One, right? If you had your choice, you'd choose Scenario One over Scenario Two 100 times out of 100.

There is only one small problem. Your choices so far have landed you in bed every Friday night of your life with yourself and a graphic novel but no peach-fragranced-body-washed angel lying next to you.

The reason you picked the wrong scenario is because you are *still* being yourself. Have you forgotten what horrible advice it is to "just be yourself"? You've heard it all your life. You've done it all your life. You are just being yourself, a total dweeb loser when it comes to women.

You are a failure on the female front when you just be yourself.

From this point forward, almost everything you do will be the opposite of what you think you should do. From this point forward you stop falling into the loser traps that you never sprang out of until you wisely got this book.

We are going to discuss the group dynamics of meeting girls in groups versus meeting them alone but the sneak-peek answer is this: yes, it's shocking but getting a phone number and date and even moving to the make-out stage and beyond that same night is far easier when she's with a group of her friends who have never in their life looked at you once unless they looked down on you. That is easier than any one-on-one in a calm, safe-feeling coffee shop.

You can still get the girl in the coffee shop. But the odds greatly decrease.

The bank robber named Willy Sutton was once asked why he robbed banks. His simple answer was, "That's where the money is."

You go to clubs and large gatherings of people to get girls because that's where lots of girls hang. And they are far more emotionally prepared to be picked up there than in the neighborhood coffee shop in the afternoon.

Note: Do you ever watch the Seinfeld reruns? George Costanza (almost a perfect twin in his character to my George Pilkington!) decides absolutely nothing he ever does gets the girl. Jerry explained it well: "If every instinct you have is wrong... then the opposite would have to be right!" George decided to do the opposite of the instincts that every fiber of his being told him to do. The moment he met the next babe, he told her he was a loser: "I'm unemployed and I live with my parents." She turned toward him in a never-before seen allure that flipped his world upside down for the first time in his life and said, "Hi, I'm Victoria!" Well… in spite of Costanza's success at playing the opposite game, you need to do it differently. You will learn how to project stunning confidence (yes, you will do this when you absolutely don't have any confidence and you will find it easy to do). Admitting to being a loser doesn't work in real life; the women already know you're a loser. But it did make for a funny episode. And the concept is pretty accurate. Losers need to change everything and adopt winning characteristics if they want to move from loser to winner.

In teaching you all this magic, I am going to try to give you the "reason why it works." For example, I am going to give you the "reason why" you *will* soon be able to go up to any 10 and start talking to her no matter how difficult it is right now. I am going to give you the "reason why" getting a date with a 10 in a group of other beautiful women is easier than getting a date with her one-on-one. So keep reading.

I was lost throughout my training with George because he didn't know why it all worked and the little he did know he didn't understand the importance of teaching me the "reason why" behind it all. As George spent the weeks following our night at Carlos's Pies teaching me how to do what he did, I devoured other resources that until that moment I didn't know existed. I'll leverage all that work for you. I'll not only teach you *what to do* but the *why you do it*. I believe you will be more successful when you don't question every nuance the way I did.

10
THE RESOURCES YOU MUST HAVE

I assure you that if you follow my advice that appears between now and the final page of this book you will get the women. Still, there is no way I can teach you the ins and outs of all the strategies or answer all your questions here. I am going to give you the blueprint you need but if you then want to take it to the next level of skill you should do some research. Fortunately, you don't have to do a lot. I did a lot and found that the following four resources are *all you need*.

They consist only of: two books, a TV show, and an audio series.

By the time you finish this book, you'll walk into clubs and other places where girls are and walk out with a beauty some of the time, and walk out with their phone number *all* of the time. But if you want to be *even better* don't question it, just get these resources and study them too, in this order:

1. *The Game*

    The Game is a book written by Neil Strauss and is considered the *first resource to be read by any guy wanting to learn about getting a girl.* (Actually, *this book* is now the real first source anyone should read! It's a far better into for fanboys like us.) *The Game* reads like a story but is non-fiction. *The Game* produced countless other resources out there and brought *Game* – as it's known – to the masses.

It is a highly interesting book and shows the author's real-life progression from loser to player. Yep, similar in concept to this one, but Neil was far cooler than I ever was even pre-Game before Neil was cool he was far more than me. In spite of it being an excellent overview, his book is not a how-to manual as much as this one is, but *The Game* does show many concepts.

Warning: Do *not* get the abridged audio book version. It omits not only key "reason why" concepts but also background tactics and makes the resulting abridgement convoluted. Read the full book to get all the charts and details.

Another reason to read this book first, besides the fact that EVERY player is supposed to (for good reason), is that it introduces you to Mystery. Mystery, aka Erik von Markovik, is the true king and modern-day producer of the fundamental PUA materials. Without Mystery, countless men would have spent countless nights all alone the past decade or more. *The Game* actually doesn't always portray Mystery in the best light; he has some emotional issues in the book. But Mystery never seemed to mind *The Game* being published and *The Game* certainly has been financially rewarding to Mystery because it set up tens of thousands of newcomers to Game and created a hungry audience of males willing to get Mystery's own materials that came later. Speaking of Mystery (Erik von Markovik):

2. *The Mystery Method – How to Get Beautiful Women in Bed*

The Mystery Method is your next must-get resource, a book written by the man himself, Mystery. This book gets into the nitty-gritty of Game using charts and a 3-tiered system, each tier with its own three parts, that you have to master. Fortunately, it's pretty fun to master because every time you learn the next of the nine pieces you get more and more (and more and more…) girls along the way.

Do not short-cut this book! Study the charts and when Mystery teaches you things like A1 and M3 (these are two of the nine parts). *Learn it.*

This volume's technical aspects are critical for you to learn. Now if you learn how to implement the nine parts but don't learn their code-name references such as *A2*, you can get all the girls you want but later in the fourth resource that I insist you get, you won't know what they are talking about when they refer to specifics such as *A2*. So pay attention to these details when you first read and study *The Mystery Method.*

3. *The Pick-Up Artist* double-season TV show (Be certain to watch Season One first!)

This is a reality show where each season begins with a group of guys just like you and me: losers. Each week, Mystery and his trained helpers teach the crew a new Game technique. Each week you watch these losers turn from loser to winner. And each week, Mystery eliminates one of the losers who just didn't cut it.

You see the real guys in action, watching how Mystery and his crew walk into a room and walk through scores of better-looking guys and within seconds they have the rapt attention of the best-looking women there, and within a minute or two they're making out. Yeah, it's a little crass there but you will still be amazed when you see it. Its purpose is to show the guys competing in the show that all this stuff is not only possible, but it is *very* possible.

And Mystery is no great shakes in the looks department. That has nothing to do with his success. And fortunately, it had nothing to do with mine. Or yours.

You will fast-forward in your training as you watch these shows. You can watch them back to back on Amazon's on-demand video and probably on Netflix, etc. But once you've finished this book and then completed the two book resources I listed above, you *need this show to help reinforce everything you have learned to this point.* In watching the losers, I mean the contestants, mess up and begin to get things right eventually, you will find that you are less likely to make the same mistakes as often.

4. *The Mystery Method Interview Series* – Multi-Volumes

The Mystery Method Interview Series is an audio course that runs 20 volumes. Google around because you might be able to locate a complete set for less than the cost of them individually from Amazon.

The Mystery Method Interview Series is the *cornerstone* of all your knowledge! *The Mystery Method Interview Series* is the deepest training you will receive in Game. It sky-rockets your skills to heights unimaginable before.

Why not just start there? Because The Mystery Method Interview Series assumes you already know the basics. The Mystery Method Interview Series assumes you know about Neil Strauss's book, that you understand Mystery's A1-A3 series, and that you understand concepts such as "body rocking" that you never fully understand the power of until you see it on Mystery's TV show.

Lest you think I have some hero-worship for Mystery (and I do admire the man and I am *so* grateful he laid the groundwork for us getting laid) this audio course does not at any time use Mystery! It was produced by a set of protégées and friends and partners of Mystery.

This course is as deep as a university course would be. Each volume in this series is devoted to how to approach a women, how to escalate from non-touch to kissing, how to *number close* (get her phone number), and so on. These audios provide you with a foundation that cannot be rocked out from under you by any hot 10 in the universe.

If you choose to keep your skill-set at this book, and one to three of the above resources, you'll be getting laid by the next Comic-Con you attend too. But if you want to be a *pro* at Game, you are absolutely lacking if you do not get and listen to every volume of *The Mystery Method Interview Series*.

Simplicity: go ahead and order as many of these as you can currently afford. You'll master this book's material about the time Amazon gets the first one in your mailbox and you'll be ready for it then.

Note: Be sure and "do" these resources in the order I've listed above. You absolutely must read *The Game* before you read *The Mystery Method – How to Get Beautiful Women in Bed* before you watch *The Pick-Up Artist* before you ratchet your skills up to pro-level with *The Mystery Method Interview Series*.

An extra bonus: By the time you've finished Mystery's book, the second resource above, you should begin reading a guy named Roissy. His blog, or at least many of his posts in a blog, is here: http://heartiste.wordpress.com/. I suggest click to read his blog archives first. In other words, go to the very earliest post he ever made and read them in order from the start until now.

11
STEP-BY-STEP – BE A HUMAN COMPUTER IN ORDER TO BE A STUD

As much as I want to get away in this book from my back-and-forth conversations with George both at Carlos's Pies and then during the weeks following that evening, I need you to know one more thing about what he taught me at the very beginning.

That fateful night as George started telling me how he transformed from a loser geek to a player who couldn't beat the women off him long enough to get a free moment to himself, my disbelief-radar was certainly up. My spider-sense was constantly on the verge of tingling but I knew sitting there at Carlos's that George was telling me the truth. Every. Single. Word.

That night for the first time since I knew him George was different.

He was just as pudgy. His hair was slightly different, sort of mussed up more than usual but still clean. His clothes were as clean as always except he didn't tuck his T-shirt all the way in; it was sort of half tucked on one side and hanging low on the other. Such a dweeb. (This was my first thought. I *now* understand he did that only after careful planning. Alpha Males have far too much on the ball to worry about every clothing detail although they certainly always look good given their selection.)

He had some of his brother's idiotic gaudy rings and a huge gold watch and a thick chain around his neck but otherwise I couldn't put my finger on anything big that was different about him. Except his manner. George was George but he was not George.

Even Though This Actually Happened to George, It Couldn't Ever Happen to Me!

In my group of four close friends, I was the ringleader. I was the star (until now). I had more confidence than they did. George was a distant second-place in the confidence category. Enzo and Frank were a far-away third and fourth place but still cool.

Not really cool, but cool as defined by George and me. Meaning, not-so-cool really but all were my faithful companions who loved all the things I loved and couldn't get a girl any better than I could.

After George had talked for 45 minutes or so, my mouth was probably hanging open with drool was coming out the sides. I mean the world as I knew it had just turned upside-down and inside-out. George was getting women. A lot of them. Beautiful ones. And he said it was solely because *he learned how*. And he said it had nothing to do with having any confidence. That is a good thing since we had none in the female arena. You will soon see that it has everything to do with *projecting* confidence. But you can pull this off without really having confidence which is the saving grace for guys like us.

As George finally took a pause and drank a sip of Coca-Cola, I said, "George this is the most unreal thing I could have ever imagined. No, I *never* could have imagined you would be sitting here telling me this stuff."

"I have Rick to thank. A lot of this stuff comes naturally to him. A lot of this stuff he did without thinking which is why everybody, girls and guys, always like my brother so much. But when he moved to Maine, Rick met some guys who told him about Game. [If you skipped through the last chapter's resource list because you wanted to get to the meat of this book, shame on you. You need to go back because there are terms there I described that you now need to know. While there, order those resources!] And although Rick realized a lot of Game came naturally to him, it didn't *all* come naturally and he learned some of the more advanced stuff."

George went on. "When I got to Rick's and broke down like the miserable little loser lizard I was when he asked about my girlfriends, Rick knew enough about Game at that point to be able to teach me the basics. I didn't believe him because I thought he was just Rick and everything in life comes easy to him. But I learned, most things in life come easy to Rick *solely because of Game. Solely because he naturally does what I learned to do and what you can learn to do.*"

I pondered what he said.

No way though.

"George, look I believe you. I believe every word you told me. And although I have 1,000 questions racing through my mind right now, like how do I learn to do all this and also questions like, *What's it like being with a shirtless, braless girl man? Do they feel as good as they look?? And Yeah, have you had sex yet??? And do you realize I'm almost two decades old and I haven't even kissed one yet????*"

"But George," I went on, "before you continue and before I give you a dump truck full of questions, I want to say this: I don't see it happening to me."

"You're the better of the two of us!" George countered. "You can do this way better than I'll ever be able to."

"I don't see it George."

"Did you ever watch that TV show called *Monk*?" he asked.

"The 'defective detective'? Yea."

"Well, he got married and if *he* can get laid so can you."

"It was a TV show goofbag!"

"Doesn't matter. The idea is accurate."

"But Monk couldn't even *talk* to women. He couldn't hold a conversation with one he liked if he tried, especially those years of have extreme OCD after his wife died."

"Monk is *exactly* a perfect example of someone who needs Game. He can't do anything on his own but if he's given a script and told to follow the instructions exactly, then he's in his perfect environment. *You* can't talk to women either but you can follow a script I give you and move and stand exactly as I tell you to. If you do that, you'll get laid."

That was crazy. I wanted to believe it. I didn't. But I did because George had done it successfully. But I didn't believe it too. (You know what I mean. You're thinking all those things too about yourself.)

George finally asked, "How long have you written programs for computers?"

"As long as I can remember," I told him.

"All you have to do is that. Be a computer. I can give you the step-by-step instructions of what to do, what to say first, second, and third to a girl. I will tell you when to move and how to move. I will tell you exactly when you praise her and exactly when to turn your back on her and start talking to someone else."

"I can't talk to strange women George!"

"You can't talk to *any* women you idiot!"

(He had a point.)

"But you can follow instructions, especially if you practice the steps. I can give you a flowchart, heck I can write it in pseudo code, and you can follow the code."

He went onto explain that's all I do. Step 1, stand this way. Step 2, say this. Step 3, say that. Step 4, move this way. Step 5, touch her friend this way.

"That's all well and good if she responds the way you say she will but what if she says something that's not in your programmed script?!"

George looked at me calm and cool and replied, "That's the whole beauty of everything. If the girl says something that doesn't fit it doesn't matter. If she says something unexpected to a question, as long as she has a congruent tone it doesn't matter what she says! You don't even have to listen to her words. You just keep following the program man."

George went on: "Last night I was at Pete's [Pete's is a new club on the other side of town, extremely popular which means I'd never been there]. I moved to the back of Pete's to meet this hot girl who was sitting with two other women and I was three minutes into our conversation before the music died down enough for me to hear *one word she said!*"

George, calm and collected, continued, "Look, she had her hand on my knee and was turned looking and talking only to me by the time I literally heard one word she had said to that point! She and I came back here to Carlos's 20 minutes later and had a couple of slices at that table right over there. I then took her home where we made out in my car *for 30 minutes at her insistence* before she went inside and but not before she told me that if I didn't call her today she'd kill me."

I have to admit, the proof is in the pudding.

Wow.

"As much as I need exactly what you are telling me here, why aren't you with her instead of me?"

"What do you mean?" George asked.

"When you called her today, didn't you set up another date?"

"I didn't call her. I don't plan to call her at least for 2 or 3 days. And maybe never."

I am staring at my best friend but I didn't know him anymore.

Seriously, realization sank in fast. Everything I knew about women was a lie. And everything I knew about George would never be the same again.

I was staring at my friend George but looking at a god.

12
A MUST-DO FIRST STEP:
PEACOCKING

Your class begins now.

Peacocking

I assure you this is one thing you must do but will not want to do. You will resist me. I've been in your shoes. I know.

You must change your appearance. Now.

You like the way you look, right? Not to sound like a broken record, but again, how have things been working out for the past few years on the girl front?

Peacocking is the term used for changing your appearance. Doing so will produce far better results at Game. There are no hard and fast rules to peacocking. But if you dress well, or if you dress the way most good-looking guys on average do, then you need to change now!

If you're like me, you don't dress the way most good-looking guys do. You're a geek so you either make the *grave* mistake of wearing shirts with mutants or hobbits on them or you blend in with all the other "nice guys" who never get girls, as I've said before, you tuck your ironed Polo in, your hair is in place, and so on.

The guy who walks into a club and leaves with the best-looking girl does not look like a geek and he does not look like the average good-looking guy there. He stands apart from the crowd. In a busy, loud environment of a club or anywhere such as a fairly empty grocery store, something you do that is showy gets you attention. If you don't fuss with whatever it is and as long as you can get it out of your geek head that you've got something on your body you never would have had a month ago, it will sit there on you and do its job. That means it does part of your job for you.

The more things we can stack on your to-do list, and the more steps of the computer program we're calling here picking-up girls (good name, huh?) you can automate, the less chance you will be yourself and the bigger chance you will leave with a female who is not your mom or sister.

It Doesn't Take Much but It Takes Something

So what can you do to peacock? First, untuck your polo or Tee. Sort of half tuck in part of it and don't worry about it. Take a shower before going out and wash your hair but don't get every hair in place. Or get it all in place and then get a blow dryer and mess it up a little. Get the wind-blown look and then don't worry about it. Look at any Esquire magazine and ignore the ads with obvious homosexuals and look at the casual wear ads. (Okay, they're all probably homosexuals but the ads are helpful to you.) Notice the guys are confident, *smiling*, and have a relaxed look at all times.

Now you need something else. Perhaps a strange hat. Not a baseball cap or anything typical. Something unique. Actually, if you go to a cowboy-themed club a baseball cap isn't necessarily wrong because it differentiates you but such a cap is so typical and there are many other things you can do to distinguish yourself.

Whatever you pick, whether a hat or chains or gaudy jewelry or a wild shirt or you grow a goatee, it does not have to reflect anything about your personality. Why would you want to be yourself, the girl doesn't want *you*! She wants someone who is willing to go out on a limb clothing-wise and not care but be confident. It cannot be too far out for the situation, you just have to do it and forget it.

For a club, you could do what is simplest. It's what I've said that Rick did naturally and now George his brother does on purpose: wear big, gaudy gold rings, watches, and a chain or two around your neck. If you're among a bunch of Jersey boys who are doing the same, *obviously you don't do that.* Be smart. If it's a cowboy-themed club go urban. (And not Urban Cowboy!) If it's a modern club atmosphere go cowboy as much as you can stomach it. Or at least wear the hat and boots. Just do something that makes you stand apart from all others there. No, you don't wear an orange jumpsuit perhaps but what you do can be somewhat extreme based on what the average guy in the room does.

Why Peacocking is Critical

Women are strongly attracted to confident men. It's an unconscious thing and they are attracted to such men because they want and need to be protected. A confident man can take her by the hand and protect her. He can guide her. Women want guidance. (I strongly urge you to read the following book for proof and for a blueprint on how to pull it off: *How to get Almost Instant Obedience from Your Woman.*)

You need all the help you can get in the confidence department, right? Dressing differently from others, setting yourself apart, is one way to project confidence even when you don't feel it. It is the goal of this book to make you project the strong confidence you do not feel. It means you follow things as outlined here without thought. When you over-think things, such as planning to walk up to a hot girl to ask her out the past 5 years but never did, the simple reason you never did is because you over-thought it and talked yourself out of it.

You need help.

Peacocking first catches the eye of the women in a place. Men don't notice what people wear. Women *always do.*

Do something different, from wearing a strange and unique hat, to the gaudy jewelry, to actually wearing a feather boa around your neck!

Note: Mystery's favorite peacocking tool – when he first begins talking to a chick who's a 10 – he removes his boa and puts it around her neck and says, "Hang onto this, it looks good there, I'll be back to get it in a sec" and then he might turn away and talk to one of her friends in the group. This is a *lock-in prop,* it tells the girl he trusts her with something and she really can't go too far because she's waiting for the retrieval. Mystery eventually gets back to it and sort of uses it to lasso her closer to him as he escalates the touch. A lock-in prop helps cement her to you. It might even be your hat you stick on her head or anything like that. But we're getting way too far too fast here and I'll lose you because you will begin thinking, *I can't do any of that man!* before you've begun. So we'll come back to things like that.

For now, just know you need an eye-catcher which means you must stand out somehow. If you think a unique hat or neck chains are overboard, you're wrong. You *could* go overboard with peacocking such as walking in looking like a pimp, but you probably will under-do it if anything. So don't be afraid to try two or three things.

The great thing about women is their sheer number! You will be going out and meeting so many that you will be able to *calibrate* what you do over time. You will learn to read them and test yourself against past attempts and learn what peacocking items work better than others. But that is down the road. I cannot tell you strongly enough how important peacocking is. It gets her attention on *you* long before you put any attention on her. If you do not do this, you make your *approach* – the term for first meeting her – far more difficult than it has to be.

Note: Remember, probably you will underdo your peacocking accessories so decide on something and then do one step further or add one more item. Later you'll calibrate such things to know that more or fewer things work.

More About Why Peacocking is Required

The peacocking accessories you use, or the way you dress differently, is often called *chick bait*. When something about you is different, all the women's eyes go to that and to you. This in no way gets you the woman; if only it was so easy. But it is one thing on a stack of other things you are going to do that will all sum up to those 9's and 10's that win you over to her.

The only skill related to peacocking that you must master is to learn to ignore your peacocking item(s). If you dwell on them and wonder if they look silly, they will. If you ignore them then you project the image of a guy who stands out, knows it, and is fully confident enough to pull it off.

Tip: If you have to, dress up with your peacocking and drive to the next town over where you don't know anyone. Walk around, go to Wal-Mart, get a Starbucks. Be self-confident about the peacocking and get it out of your system. Later when you eventually end up in the venue you are going to meet a woman you won't focus so much on your accessories. And there's a chance a female will show interest in the other town. Like a dog who chases cars, you won't know what to do with her when you get her through your peacocking alone, but it will give you good feedback of how well it works.

Peacocking not only gets her attention, it tells her you are confident when you aren't. I mean who in their right mind would wear huge gold rings and a thick chain necklace? My friend George does and he gets laid. You don't and you don't.

You know the jerks you've seen who are goofy around women, look silly, but still they smile and talk loudly to them and don't care how they look? They get far more babes than you. Because although they lack lots of skills they project an "I-don't-care" confidence and that is somehow – we don't have to understand it, just accept it – somehow that is a magnet to women.

10's and 9's!

I'll come back to this a lot, but if you try these things to approach 5's, 6's, 7's, and 8's, you not only are getting an inferior female but you also will not have as much success. Those girls are so under-confident themselves, they start second-guessing things that winner girls don't second-guess.

The 9's and 10's have their radar up always on the lookout for someone who is actually different from the 1,000 boys each year who approach them and look the same and say the same old stupid things.

Your Smile Goes with the Peacocking

Rick taught George a trick and he taught it to me.

You have *got to be smiling* when you enter a room with girls.

You have *got to be smiling* when you start the pick-up tactics I show you below.

But you don't feel like smiling because you'll be so frightened. So do this: When you adorn your peacocking item(s), for example, you put on that red vest that you wouldn't have been caught dead in before, put on your smile. The *smile* has to be connected to your peacocking item so consciously smile and keep it up when you put on your vest or hat or paint your nails black or whatever you do to be different. Do this when you're home where you're comfortable and able to smile.

Tip: If you have a favorite stand-up comedian who makes you laugh, get some MP3s or videos and listen and/or watch as you dress to go out. It'll get you in a mood you need to be in; a smiling, friendly, and more relaxed mood. If it's a cynical comedian so much the better because it will help you adopt a don't-care attitude which is icing on the cake to get a woman.

Note: A primary foundational truth is that don't-care attitudes attract women and showing interest in her repels her. Let me remind you again that you know nothing about women. If you walk into a yard full of cats, the one cat you want to pet will be the one that runs away from you every time you bend down to her. The way you get to pet that cat is to ignore it and work the rest of them, looking at and talking to and petting all the others when they let you. The one you ignore will make a beeline straight to you when she realizes you don't want to pet her. I cannot express how much females are just like that. It is almost impossible for you to believe right now, but as you will see the very first time you try these skills, a don't-care, friendly to everyone-else confident-enough-to-dress-any-darn-way-I-please attitude gets the one you ignore most. (If she's a 9 or 10. They are not used to being ignored. If *they*, the best in the house, are ignored it does two things: It knocks them down a notch and it bumps you up a notch. They don't know how to handle guys who show little initial interest and they go crazy trying to get his attention and attraction. Like the cat you don't go for, the 9 or 10 is attracted to your avoidance like bugs to a nightlight. If you are not all ga-ga over her, you must be some stud! This *is* the way she thinks and even she is not usually aware this is happening.)

Mystery likes to look somewhat Goth. Yeah, that is stupid to the uninformed but the reason it works is because he *never* goes where Goth people go. He's the only one in the place with black nails. And he smiles and wears both his smile and his black nails and his idiotic-looking tall Dr. Seuss-like hat and his boa with ease only because he consciously doesn't think about his peacocking and he smiles the moment he gets into his Goth things. So he walks into a *normal* club where every guy is normal and the women immediately look at him and nobody else. And he is calm and smiling and the girls have no idea why but they want to know this guy to see if he can keep their mental curiosity as well as he grabbed their eye curiosity by his peacocking. He does get the women. He gets the 10s. Most of the time he says absolutely nothing that detours from the script you'll learn below.)

But I'm Fat, Thin, Bald, Hairy…

Women are as shallow as we are but in different ways.

Yes, women are attracted to good-looking guys but it's not an attraction that does much to get the good-looking guys very far. As for what we men want, if she doesn't remind us of our mom, then there's a chance we'll want to date her if she would have us. (This will change quickly as your success with women grows exponentially in the next few weeks. You will not settle for second-best ever again.)

If you are a confident smiling guy who is so care-free you peacock and not think twice about it and if you are also bald or fat then you are *just as attractive* to a 9 or 10 whom you ignore than if you had a bushy head of hair and a fit waistline! You might not want to sleep with someone if she's fat but women are not shallow like that. They are shallow like this: *he's ignoring me, I must be ugly and he's really got a spark I need to know more about right now.*

As long as you approach only 9's and 10's this will work miracles for your bedtime. You must trust me. I am proof and George is *double* proof.

How Does One Peacock at Comic-Com?

I was pretty good at Game before I went to Comic-Con. As I said earlier, I hadn't yet slept with a woman but that was only because I had no place to do so. Sure, I could have gotten a hotel but it just didn't seem right each time. But I had everything but the lay before Comic-Con. In my car, in theirs, in club bathrooms, behind Pete's, and other places.

It was always my plan, sort of, to meet a girl at Comic-Con and get 'er done there. I figured what a coup! For *me* to get laid in the first place would be a modern marvel. For *me* to get laid while attending Comic-Con would be an achievement that could not be beat. Not only do guys who go to Comic-Con not get laid, they *certainly* don't get laid while attending the convention!

Yet, I was getting good and my only problem was this: would there even be enough single 9's and 10s at Comic-Con to pull this off?

If you've been the Comic-Con you know that the majority of guys and girls are traditional geeks: fat, bald, ugly, pompous (for some odd reason, we fans develop a strong sense of sarcasm and haughtiness over others; I think it's a self-protection thing because if we didn't have that we'd have *nothing*).

But if you have been to Comic-Con or seen videos about it on the 'Net, then you know there are tons of people there, from movie studios to artists to fans to stars to hundreds and hundreds of people working the booths to wait staff at all the food places around and so on. 90% of the people there are losers. (Like us. You can get angry and stop now but you know I am speaking truth.)

So many people are at Comic-Con though that the other 10% who are not losers comprise a very large number indeed! I figured there would two or three hundred 9's and

10's there, half or more who would not be married or attached strongly to someone else.

I had a chance. By that time I had been going after only the best-looking woman in the club, coffee shop, school function, restaurant, or wherever else I found myself.

But I'm getting a little ahead of myself bragging too much.

The focus here is this: How does anyone peacock at Comic-Con where every other idiot walking around has some costume, make-up, light-making hammer or shield or light saber, or hobbit ears, or a wizard wig?

I certainly would not go in costume. If I did I would be just another loser.

The guys who go to Comic-Con who aren't in costume dress like I used to, tucked-in Polo, etc. Or worse, wearing character T-shirts.

If I say so myself, my choice of peacocking attire was perfect and could not be outdone by anyone, not even Mystery. I would go in an expensive suit and tie! I would have a gold watch and 4 non-gaudy gold rings on. (They are each fake but they look good and rich!)

I would peacock – I would stand apart from *everybody there* – by dressing like the 50,000 businessmen downtown in San Diego that day. But at Comic-Con I would be the cock of the walk! Nobody would come close. Nobody would be dressed like me.

And the proof is in the pudding. I got laid. And as I was getting laid, I still had all four rings on and my button down shirt was unbuttoned but still on and still looking good!

Use this as an example. Use your imagination; think outside the box. Wherever you plan to go to meet girls think through the best way to peacock and make the most of that venue.

Note: In today's way-too-casual world, dressing up in a suit, or at least casual-formal, will make you peacock like no other when just a few years ago it wouldn't be unusual. Again, in a business setting, if you work for a corporation for example, dressing in a suit and tie at work doesn't get you noticed but in today's world just about everywhere it does. If you truly are at a loss for what to do and you do not trust me that something gaudy like a big gold chain won't do it (it works great when you project confidence you don't really feel) (and I'll show you exactly how to do just that) then dress up man! I recently flew to see my Uncle in Texas and I dressed in a suit and tie just to peacock since it worked well at Comic-Con. Everybody treated me with respect and with far more courtesy than they ever do otherwise. I'm just a kid still in many ways, or I feel that way at least. I learned that today, a suit is more than clothing; it also demands instant honor and respect. The suit is an under-utilized peacocking sensation. Just don't go polyester in the suit or tie! Look at Joseph A. Bank's website and catalogs and go with the trend there and you'll have ladies seeing you far sooner than you see them. And for Alpha Males that is exactly the way it is supposed to work.

13
YOUR APPROACH

Have you ever shot a gun? I live in Arizona. Yes, I've shot a gun. A lot of them. If you don't like that then if you ever see me in person, tell me that you don't like people to shoot guns. Then if someone tries to harm us or rob us I promise you that I will not offend your sensibilities and save your life.

Anyway. What was I talking about?

Oh yes.

We Arizonians can often shoot accurately with a rifle or handgun that is not malfunctioning or adjusted wrongly. The reason it is so difficult to hit a bulls-eye is because:

1. New shooters have no confidence

2. New shooters don't follow the simple order of proper shooting

3. New shooters add to the aim, strain too much, and do far more than they are supposed to.

So they miss. A good shooter doesn't add to or take away from the extremely simple rules for hitting the target.

A *PUA* (pick-up artist) knows this too.

If you want to success, you will peacock and then do exactly what I tell you to do. If you do more, and if you improvise any step, you will fail.

The hard part is going to be just doing what I tell you and no more.

This is where the TV Show I told you to watch, *The Pick-Up Artist*, comes in handy. Because by the time you start watching it in the next week or two or three, you will know a lot of these concepts. Hopefully you will have practiced on your own in private.

You will fail for a while anyway because when you first start you'll forget things, you'll skip a step, and you'll improvise. *The Pick-Up Artist* will show guys who know less than you will know when you start watching them. You will see how difficult it is for them to follow just these two rules:

1. Smile

2. Never directly look at a woman you're talking to.

You will see the guys on the show fail every time they fail those two simple instructions. By seeing their failures I believe you can avoid most of your training mistakes. I know this because I was fortunate enough to have watched the show the very week I began going out testing these skills. By seeing the guys on the show mess up somehow it helped me not to. I was able to follow the plan fairly well. So much so that on my first night out I left with a hot chick's phone number.

(Keep in mind, I basically had never before that night *talked* to a woman hotter than a 7.)

Jerks and Jerk-Offs

Do you ever feel this way:

Jerks get the women while nice guys stand around wondering "what just happened?"

I don't want you to feel extremely bad but the truth is that this statement is a fact.

You are going to have to take women off the pedestal you've put them on ever since puberty. You have *got* to fight your every desire to be nice to them and to show them that you respect them.

You never disrespect them and you aren't to be mean to them. But there is an in-between "sweet spot" and guys who get laid, meaning most guys who are sort of jerks, get the women and you, not a jerk, just jerk-off.

Remember the cats. The kitty you show an interest in is the very one you will repel. Women do this too. It's not their fault that they *say* they want nice guys but they only *do* the jerks.

The jerks will stand up for them if they get in trouble. The nice guys might *want* to stand up to opponents but can't and won't and don't know how.

Women don't think about this but it's in their nature and you must understand it.

You Train the Woman to Respond to You with Interest

You don't have to know self-defense and be Chuck Norris to get a woman! (Being Chuck *would* help though.) You just have to learn how avoid being Mr. Nice Guy from this day forward and you have *got* to learn to shun – in a semi-subtle way – anything a hot female does that is not a direct expression of interest and desire for you. In other words, if she treats you the way they always have treated you in the past, you will punish her!

You don't punish her by hitting her or anything like that obviously. But you punish her in small, slight ways that will increase her attraction for you every time and will decrease her desire to be anything but wanting of you.

You will be doing this in the first 1 to 8 minutes of meeting her. If you do it right, you won't have to punish her much. You'll have set her up to want to know more about you. Your job won't be over after the 8 minutes but you will have gotten past the hard part.

Sound Like an Impossibility? Here's is How You Will Do It

You will do all of this automatically. You will be following the script. You will stand how I say and say what I tell you to say.

Isn't that a relief? Like me, you can follow a script as long as you don't have to come up with something to say to the girl, right? Just say what I tell you to say, and don't think about it.

Literally, I will tell you exactly how to walk up to her and what to say. Practice a few times. Then you can do it. It *is* that easy.

And now that you know to peacock at home before you leave, your programming in front of your first girl appears now with *the approach*.

The Approach

The approach is a term for the first time you speak to a particular girl.

Where do you go the first time you try the next few tactics you learn here? You go where the most hot girls are.

I strongly urge you to pick the best place in your town for your first night out. This is the hottest club in town. Yes, this means even if you never been to a club in your life. And if a line forms and bouncer only lets certain people in after it gets busy you will have to arrive early to get in and you'll just hang out until it gets hopping. This way you don't fight the line, the wait, and the bouncer who limits who can go in next, often letting the cool people he knows and the hot girls in and guys like us stand in line until closing time.

By the way, you might fail your first night out as green as you will be. But "fail" is success now. Fail in this context means you won't get many words and actions out before the girl you're trying to meet quits talking to you and moves to another area and ignores you.

Still, you have succeeded! You must believe me man! After 3 or so times, you will have gotten way past *approach anxiety* on your very first night! Ta-da, that was the hardest part! Everything else gets easier. If you can't approach then nothing else matters as proved by your life the past few years. That is all going to change now! So plan to go out and approach 4 or 5 women. Hot women, it only all works on them. If you can approach, just *open* them (meaning simply start a conversation) you will go home and recall your success for the first time perhaps and the next night you'll get further.

You will come home higher than a cocaine addict on speed.

You may not be at Comic-Con and get laid your first night out but you will be *on your way* there!

But you *might* get far the first night. Because who knows, you might really be a natural PUA. If all you can't to is approach and open a girl, you'll be past that. Once she starts talking to you and once she zeroes in on whatever you peacock with and once you get her attention unlike every other guy in the room, you *might* just let nature take its course.

My suspicion? If you're like me, you will need far more to get past the approach. But who knows? The breakthrough might very well come faster for you than for most of us.

Your First Goal Reviewed

Probably, you can't do an approach. So night one, your only goal is to do an approach three or four times with three or four *targets*. (The target is the 9 or 10 you want to talk to next.)

You need to go to a club where lots of people are. The places we geeks always hated (until we see how quickly they become the primary source for all the tang we can handle).

If You Must Arrive Early

As mentioned above, if you are going to a busy club you may to arrive early. If so, you really don't want to drink too much. It's fine and almost certainly best if you drink *no alcohol at all the entire night.*

Just order a club soda and nurse it.

Body language plays a huge role in all this as you will see in the rest of this book. Girls read body language like the latest gossip column and men have no clue about body language.

You will definitely feel the need to hold your drink up at chest level as you walk around. *Don't do this!* You are putting up a shield between you and the skirt and she will notice this subconsciously. She will sense you have confidence issues and it hurts you to hold your drink there. Yet think about it – we all do this.

Stop now. Even at home or any time you carry a glass, from now on practice carrying it the way a confident Alpha Male carries it; low, almost at your thigh level, sort of holding it as an afterthought. The body language you portray this way tells women you are open and fearless. I know, this is a silly thing but it's true. Lots of these things you are learning seem silly and many are microscopically helpful. Yet they all add up to that magic number 10 you are hoping to get a date with.

Smile Man, Smile!

My advice on smiling the moment you peacock while still at home is so important, it's worth mentioning again. You are *not* to walk around that club or anywhere else from now on without a smile on your face. Fake it man, fake it!

You'll quickly learn that you are doing it automatically. That will help once you get to the club. So start doing it now. Don't even wait to be peacocking, start now and whether it's your Mom or Dad, sister or brother, neighbor, teacher, or cop, you smile as you walk down the street, as you enter a place, as you get out of your car, as you order at restaurants.

You can be absolutely perfect at Game doing everything else correctly, standing properly, holding your drink low, and saying every word confidently and if you do not smile the women will not be drawn to you nearly as much. Why not get in this all-important habit now?

Tip: In as many of these techniques as you can, begin implementing them in your life everywhere you go, not just to clubs. The sooner you do this the better you will be when you face a 9 or 10 and the less you'll have to think about. I wish George knew to give this advice to me, I learned it later in some of the resources I gave you earlier. When you walk into a coffee shop and you're the only one in there and it's just a guy behind the bar, walk up to him confidently, speak loud enough to project more than you naturally want to (you'll see why later), and smile a huge smile and maintain an I-don't-care attitude the whole time. You're just a guy out on vacation everywhere you go, or at least that's the attitude you cultivate and it cements the attitude and the smile and the voice and the tone in you for when you need it later. You will also find that the guy behind the counter gives you better service; you win even if it's around a guy. Here is why: The qualities described here are *leader qualities*. They are *Alpha Male* qualities. An Alpha Male, the leader in any group, will do all this! That is why George's brother Rick is so likable to all of us. He's a leader. But he doesn't really lead; he just projects all of these qualities I'm now teaching you. They come naturally to Rick. They don't to us. But you can add them to your personality in just a very short time. Trust me. And so when you order, even when it's just you and another guy, you are the instant leader. He doesn't know why but he looks up to you even if you're shorter! That is not a bad quality to carry through life, especially once you get out into the real world and get a real job in business. The Alpha Male gets the jobs and the promotions and is the one all others like without even knowing why.

When you are in a club, it would be great if you were the only guy there but that's not going to happen. Game requires that you be Alpha Male the moment you walk in that does *not* mean you are bigger and stronger. It means you own whatever place you step into. You own a place in other people's eyes by being confident (peacocking gets you 20% there), by projecting the proper body language, by not paying too much attention to the hot women right away, by being buddies with any guys you know, and by speaking and projecting loud enough (yes even in extremely loud clubs).

Make sure that *nobody has to ask you to repeat yourself!* Leaders speak loud enough to be heard. This doesn't mean they yell unless the music demands it but it means you are heard. You also must *speak slowly enough to be understood.* You need to begin this *now*. Smile, project your voice, and speak s-l-o-w-l-y enough to be understood. This is slower than you naturally speak by just a fraction. Practice. When you get nervous in a club you are going to speak faster than you should. By getting yourself speaking slowly and projecting *as you smile* you will ensure success later in those areas.

Above all smile. Smiling does not guarantee you woman success but the lack of one guarantees failure.

Group Dynamics Make it Far Easier

In spite of every fiber of your being that will fight me on this, let me make a simple statement that every successful PUA (Pick-Up Artist) learns extremely quickly:

It's far easier to get a 10 when she is with her friends.

I know. It makes no sense.

But you need to understand the psychology of it. She is comfortable with her friends. With women, there is safety in numbers. And the whole key is you are going after 10s and not your usual high standard of 4's and 5's.

A 10 is hit upon by guys how many times? Not in her life, *how many times this month do you think?* Everywhere she goes, guys are telling her that her eyes look pretty, her hair is nice, they love her smile, and the bolder ones express a higher interest, asking if she wants to go out before she knows his name. A 10 loves this attention but with the usual approach she just gets bored.

When 100 good-looking guys approach her in a club, if she's with her friends she can far more easily deflect them. And I did say "good-looking guys." A 10 wants something different. She wants what she doesn't have and rarely finds. She wants a guy who is worth fighting for. And that turns out to be a guy who does *not* come onto her. Good for you, because you find it easy not to be forward with women, right? But you have to do it correctly. The geek's traditional way of not showing direct interest in women doesn't work obviously.

Note: Groups are referred to as *sets*, determined by the number of women in the group. A *3-set* is a group of three females talking to each other.

If she is with a group, she will often pick women just slightly below her caliber. A 10 will be with 8.5's, 9's, and 9.5's, They all look up to the 10 and she uses them for safety in numbers. Oh, they might all like each other and be bestie friends. But unconsciously they group like this.

Normally of course the 9's are almost as hard to get as the 10. (For you and me, the 2's have been just as hard to get!) But when they group, the group dynamics give you lots of tools that work to your massive advantage:

1. You need a mechanism to get her attention by not showing her any interest *but by showing everybody else interest!* This will attract the 10 so much, it's like *chick crack.* (Hard to believe isn't it?)

2. The ones you are not targeting – her friends – are called *obstacles.* The 10 is using them to shield her from guys who will approach her that night. You will befriend all the obstacles in her group first. This works for you better because you won't be as scared to talk to them since they are not your target.

3. The 10 sees her friends talking to you. *This gives you instant status.* When she first sees you open the group, she notices that you're confidently pulling off whatever peacocking you have going for you that night. You are smiling and speaking loudly enough and slowly enough for everybody to hear. You already are better than 80% of the men who have tried to open the group. You just moved up a notch from nobody to nobody-plus, a *hard notch to get to in a 10's mind.* So you then begin opening and chatting up her friends. And the things you say *get their attention* and they start turning to you and talking to you, breaking the looking-inward circular dynamic of the group from what it was when you first approached them. The 10 then sees her friends accept you more and more as the seconds roll by! (They will. They won't feel threatened by you due to the way you stand and the things you tell them as you'll see.) Her friends will begin laughing at the things you say and probably even begin a slight touch on your arm here and there. You

have just moved up two notches from nobody-plus to possible interest by the 10.

4. Here is the key: As the initial seconds roll on, you keep chatting up her friends. *You must learn to be chatty and you'll learn how to begin developing that here.* But she awaits your noticing her because come on, she's the 10 *but you do not notice her.* And if she says anything during this initial opening time you toss a *neg* at her! A neg is a slightly negative comment. It never puts her down directly. It never is mean. A neg is a comment which at that time shows the 10 you are busy talking to her friends and she can wait in line. The common negs for this situation are, "[looking at her friends and sort of pointing to the 10 *as you smile a big grin*]We were talking here, is she always that rude?" Or, "Is she always that talkative??? You can't take her anywhere!" and then you continue the thread with the friends that you were in before the 10 said anything. You will *not lose ground* from your current status with the 10. Quite the opposite, you just *lowered her status in her own pretty little head!*

This is all so critical. You must re-read these items.

More About Why It Works

You have begun to level the playing field in a systematic manner. She started off as a 10 and you were maybe a 6 as you walked up with your peacocking and confidence. A 6 is *way* below her but still is better than average. You chatted up her friends and they accepted you. If her friends like you, being her protection group, then that automatically moves you up again to a 7 maybe 7.5. When you neg her you do not drop one notch! What happens in a neg, for 10's, is *she drops* but your status remains the same.

Note: Negging is a perfect example of why none of this works on the 6's through 8's. If you neg a girl who does not think she's a princess– because she isn't one – then she just shuts down and pouts. A 10 is *never* used to being dissed and as long as you remain happy, chatty, and smiling as you neg her and as long as you never directly put her down in a substantial way, as long as you remain playful as you neg, instead of getting angry with you – her status *drops* in her own eyes. You are still maybe a 7.5 and she just dropped a whopping full point to a 9 from the lofty 10 she was! That is closing the gap like you have never had it closed in your life and you may only be 2 minutes into the whole approach!

Easy breezy.

Without obstacles the target is far harder to hit. This goes against everything you ever would have believed before. Good, that means you are finally moving forward. The obstacles accept you. They are offering their seal of approval the more they give you attention and the more you give them attention. You are petting every cat in the group *except the one who wants to be petted the most!* The power you are beginning to possess in the group is higher than a guy has been perhaps in many weeks. And again, you're perhaps only into the set's opening 2 minutes or so!

So What Do You Specifically Do and Say to Open the Group?

The amazing thing is what you say matters very little. It's how you stand, what you project, how to say it, and your smile. Fortunately, in a loud place, what they say back to you has little bearing on what you say and do next so you don't have to stand there and break your Alpha Male building to say, "Huh?" and "What did you say?" and "Pardon me, I didn't hear you that music is too loud…"

Don't ever do that in the opening seconds of an opening. Because *what they say doesn't matter one bit. You just stay on track.* Yes, this is hard to believe until you see it work for you.

As you invest more of your time in the other resources I told you to get, you will learn lots of other openings you can use. But some guys when first learning try to get so many things in their heads they just get confused when the actual approach comes. (You'll see this on the TV show especially.)

I do think you should know about the various ways to open but I use only one opening at a time. I'll just decide on one and *use it the entire night*. And I'll have a couple of negs ready for the 10s. And I'll have a couple of interest-building stories (we'll get to that) and some kind of prop to get in the 10's hands eventually and I'll have a place to *bump* and *bounce* to and that's it. I don't load up my mind with too many things to remember.

Note: No, *bump* and *bounce* do *not* refer to things you do to her in the backseat of your car! A bounce is the term used for moving her to a different place. If you can leave the club with her and move her to get a slice of pizza close by (within walking distance is best as you build trust), and then perhaps to a less-crowded place to get another drink (you will sip yours slowly or not even drink any of it), you *speed up time* in her mind. The more places you get her to early, the more she feels like you have actually been on multiple dates. (I know, women think crazy.) Plus, by bouncing her you are creating a sense she needs to feel that she can and should follow you. This is psychologically big. A *bump* is what I call moving within the initial venue such as moving her from her group to a more private place where you begin focusing solely on her. Others have different names but I prefer bump. My bump is training for her to eventually *bounce* to a completely different building soon after.

So in this book, I am not going to give you exhaustive lists of things to say. Some websites will list tons of openings (such as http://www.pualingo.com/pua-openers/) but at this point you should learn just a couple for your first week out to get the ladies. I am also not going to give you an encyclopedia of things to say to get her bumped and bounced. I'll give you one or perhaps two. Why complicate it? She's just a female, it'll work without you overdoing things.

The 3-Second Rule

The 3-second rule was designed for guys like you and me. Chuck Norris never needed it – he never was afraid to talk to women. We need it. Still, even the expert PUAs will admit that sometimes even they are hesitant to approach women for whatever reason. Perhaps, they just got brushed off for the first time in months or some random thing turned an otherwise ordinary approach into a disaster. The 3-second rule is akin to the rule that you hear when thrown off a horse: get right back on the horse before he has a chance to walk away and more important, before *you* have a chance to walk away or the likelihood you'll ride another horse is slim

The 3-second rule says this: From the moment you see a 10, whether in a 2-set, 3-set, or #-set, you will approach the group in no more than 3 seconds. The moment you see your target, start the count-down in your head, "3... 2... 1" and by or before *1* you are opening the set.

Doing this keeps you from thinking. All of this is designed to keep you from thinking. Because if you think then the only thought will be to think yourself out of it.

Tip: I strongly suggest you don't open a girl by herself for a while. The dynamics differ from the group dynamics shown here. It's more difficult because you cannot use her friends to raise your DHV (Demonstration of Higher Value). Her friends, the obstacles, are called that because you must overcome their automatic tendency to avoid guys who approach in the common way most men approach. Here you learn to make the obstacles your friends which gives you an automatic advantage when you begin working the 10.

The rest of this book assumes you will make the 3-second rule your iron-clad rule. When you see the prize walk straight there.

Your First Opening: Body Language and the Routine

If you open without smiling, you might as well just pull out your Hulk action figure and sit in the middle of the dance floor and play "Hulk Smash!" for all the good your training will do you. Hopefully, we've covered the smile enough and you will practice it wherever you go that talking much more about it won't be necessary.

Here is the common scenario: You spot a woman, a hottie, a 9 and preferably 9.5 or 10 talking to her friends. You have your target and you see the obstacles. The 3-second rule countdown begins *now*. As the countdown begins, walk around until you can approach the group closest to the obstacle farthest from the target. The following diagram shows exactly where to make your approach and say your first thing:

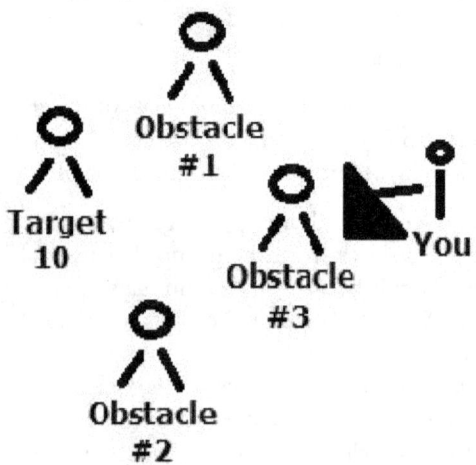

Notice you approach the obstacle farthest from the target. If it's a 2-set or a 5-set, that doesn't change. Always be the farthest away from the target so as not to make her think you're coming onto the 10. When you get near them *never ever*

face the obstacle! You pass the group by, almost bypassing all of them, wearing your confident smile, and right as you are sideways with the obstacle, you say this:

"Hey."

PUAs have used, "Hello!" and "Hi" and other short greetings but they consistently say that "Hey" works best to get the obstacle to turn and look at you. As she does, keep looking sort of at her over your shoulder in an almost sideways glance. When she does, no matter what she says or if she says nothing, just keep talking and say this:

"Did you all see those girls fighting outside???"

Don't get them a chance to respond! But just give them a moment to process what you said and continue (talking loud enough for all to hear and slowly enough for all to understand!), "Oh but get this... These girls were fighting over a guy named *Raymond!* Who would fight over a guy named Raymond?!! I bet you wouldn't!"

And as you say that, look at the next obstacle, and as you do touch her arm just for a brief moment and the remove it as you continue:

"It was knock-em, drag-em down real fighting, the whole club was out there it seemed! They were hair-pulling and clawing, and one drew blood with her nails! And this short guy was standing there just laughing... He *had* to be Raymond!"

And no matter how they respond, and you'll just be smiling and shaking your head in disbelief as you describe this girl fight, it's time to move forward. Remember, chicks for some reason are pulled towards chatty guys. You aren't chatty naturally but you are here learning a few lines and you are going to be the master at faking it.

Note: Never ever open a set with, "Can I ask you something?" You will be screaming "unconfident loser" when you do. It knocks you back down from the value your peacocking and smile gave you. Alpha Males never ask permission.

Note: Mystery likes this girl-fight opening and he goes onto say, "One of the girls' boobs popped right out for the world to see!" Your set will start smiling because they are uncomfortably thinking of themselves in that situation having a wardrobe malfunction in the midst of a huge crowd. He goes on, "And I like to see them as much as any healthy man but these were the saggy-draggy kind right out of National Geographic!"

Mystery's addition isn't a bad one as long as you practice it. Because if you *one time slow down and lose momentum during any of it, or if one of the girls asks you something and you stop to acknowledge or listen to her question, you will have blown yourself out of this set.* You are not accepted enough yet to listen to anything they have to say. You're an Alpha Male! You'll listen when you're good and ready but until then you have something funny to tell them about.

What Mystery's addition does is sort of bring up the topic of sex without bringing it up. This is good to do because it doesn't indicate you are hinting at sex. This way you discuss something like a "saggy-baggy booby" in third person and are laughing. It shows you can discuss those topics but you aren't focused on them.

An Alternative Opener

I'll give you an alternative opener below. You can practice both and I suggest you record yourself once you've practiced. As you practice and then record yourself, use your best imagination, you know the imagination you use at role-playing games with your friends... Isn't *this* role-playing more important to get right than fantasy role-playing games with the boys every Friday night?

Listen to yourself after you've practiced and record a few opening routines and determine which one is the most natural sounding. Decide which is more likely to get the set in your favor and laughing a little. Then begin with that one when you first go out. If it fails a couple of times, switch to the other and see which does better for your deliver ability.

Note: Remember, PUAs have been crafting routines for a decade and a half and tons are out there. Don't try to learn a lot of them, two are ample. But it's good to see what is there and in the resource list earlier you will find tons of routines, both for opening and then for increasing your perceived value to the set. The routines themselves are far less important than your delivery and your pulling their laughs and interest; that is done best with a winning smile and projection of confidence through your slow speaking and loud-enough, projecting voice.

Note: See, when your aunts and Mom always told you, "Just be confident, you'll find a nice girl!" the problem was they had no idea how to teach you to be confident. You are *not* confident. But now that you know what unconscious behavior confident people do, you will mimic that and others will view you as having the confidence you always wanted.

Whatever opener you decide to use first, the second can be a follow-up thread that you start saying right after you finish the first one. The next chapter explains the importance of a quick follow-up routine.

Here's a common opener that works quite well:

"Hey guys would any of you ever get a tattoo on your shoulder?"

Smiling and *body rocking* (more about this later) and projecting volume *and* speaking more slowly than you think you should. (I cannot stress the importance of this delivery. You must practice a lot before your first attempt at the club. You *can* practice *at* the club through a trial by fire, but I don't want you to get discouraged when your delivery keeps getting you shut out of the set.)

Give them slightly less time to answer than they need to the tattoo question. In other words, right as they are about to spout out whatever vapid opinion they have, just smoothly continue the routine:

"Here's why I brought it up. My 16-year old sister thinks she found the boy of her lifetime and she wants to get his name tattooed right on her shoulder!"

This time, give them just a tad longer to process and respond. After hearing she is a 16-year old they are going to begin telling you never let her do that. But don't let the set respond more than a couple or three words, and then say, "See, that's the problem! She is strong-headed and if I tell her not to, that is exactly what she wants to do more!"

As you say, "more!" reach out and touch the arm or shoulder of whichever obstacle you didn't touch before. Keep it there just a couple of seconds, about twice as long as the first touch you did earlier.

14
IMMEDIATELY START
THE NEXT ROUTINE!

If you practiced and pull off the previous chapter's opener, the girls will be laughing and saying things like, "Oh my gosh!" and when they do, you must *immediately move to your next routine!*

Note: These are all *routines*. The opener girl fight is an opening routine. Your next story is going to be a routine. You will just be chatting up a storm. As you do so, just lightly and briefly touch the arm of the next obstacle. (Recall you've already touched the arm of the one.) If this is a 3-set then you will have talked to the obstacles and touched each one by now and the 10, your target, is just standing there liking what she is seeing and hearing and beginning to miss the attention that she's used to getting when guys focus so much on her.

Do Not Square Up to any of the Girls in the Set!

Do not directly square up to an obstacle. Always sort of be facing away from the group although obviously you are going to be facing them a little more than you were when you first got their attention with "Hey!"

After you have them turned to you and you have *not* fully turned to them because you won't do that or your body language will show way too much interest too early, you will start *body rocking*. You will see this in Mystery's TV show and learn far more about its importance in the audio series I recommended but in a nutshell (and if this book is the only resource you use, you will be fine) it means that as you talk to the set you lean in and then out, towards them and then away from them as you talk. You are not a bowling pin about to fall so don't make the move dramatic. Don't be bouncy or your nervousness will be clear and you lose all status. Body rocking is more physically acting as though you only have a few seconds and not bouncing or bobbling. It's a critical move though. Its intent is to show that you absolutely like talking but there are others in the place too. You slightly lean in as you begin to talk but immediately lean out, and look elsewhere quickly a couple of times as you speak. Don't look elsewhere like you are running from the law; it's just that you're the Alpha Male and you like to know what is going on.

You do ultimately square yourself up to a female, either the obstacles or, ultimately, your target. Once the whole set, one or more obstacles, or your target begin showing interest in you, you can reward them by turning toward them. This helps reinforce their good behavior. Don't stay that way though, it's just a short reward for good behavior such as an *IOI*.

An IOI is an *Indicator of Interest*. A girl shows IOIs by:

- Touching her face as she looks at you (you didn't know this, did you? Look for it, it's a powerful IOI that indicates she likes you so far)

- Unconsciously touching/twisting/playing with her hair as she looks at you

- Looks you over and not with a critical eye

- Talks with you when you are momentarily quiet (which you won't be much in the opening two routines especially)

- Smiles and laughs *genuinely* at what you say (you know the difference between placating you and a genuine response. Be honest, but truly if you practice and are chatty, enthusiastic, and smile, most of their smiling and laughing responses *will* be genuine)

- She gives you a compliment

- Touching you in some way

- She holds eye contact well and obviously willingly

- Buys you a drink

- She asks you a question (multiple questions are exceptionally high IOIs) (asking if you have a girlfriend is da bomb!) (You never answer directly; you could say, "Doesn't everybody?" and move on with your next routine.)

As soon as you see an IOI, turn to her. If it's an obstacle, it just gets your foot into the door of the set faster. By the way, if she disagrees with you but in a playful, laughing way, that is an IOI! If she punches your arm but laughs and is playful that is an IOI! Don't toss away your brain throughout all this in spite of our attempt to automate as much as possible for you at this point.

Note: Beginning Gamers often ask here, "What if the obstacle really starts liking me?" Keep her in mind for later in the target doesn't work out. Rules were made to be broken but not often and this obstacle has got to be someone amazing that you mis-calculated before entering the set for you to move on her when she was never the original target. If you mis-read her IOIs and drop the 10 for nothing, you will be blown out of the set quickly. It's best to stick to your original plan and keep targeting the 10.

So you square up to reward their behavior but otherwise you'll always be slightly askew, looking around (body rocking), never bouncing, smiling, enthusiastic, glad to be there and to be seen. Again, don't over-emphasize your enthusiasm or you will become someone who is watching the place instead being the calm, cool guy that all the others are watching.

The opposite of an IOI is an *IOD*, an *Indicator of Disinterest*. This happens if she frowns or slightly looks away from you. If it's an obstacle, you turn to another obstacle and continue. If it's the target, you have to toss her a neg. Say this, "Hey, I like your hair and it would look even better up [say down if it's already up]."

You can also punish an IOD by turning away from them and immediately interacting with another person, especially if it's another person in the set. Always punish an IOD but don't show any disappointment or pouting. You're Alpha Male! Just turn away from it without changing your smile and certainly don't show her you noticed the IOD. If you are able to turn your back completely to her right after she tosses you an IOD (again, whether an obstacle or later even the target) you have dramatically punished her. Women do *not* like that and unconsciously they will learn quickly not to react so negatively to you.

Shit Tests

Some IODs are *shit tests* which is the term used for tests women toss at you and all other men to see if you are the real thing or a phony. You're a phony but you will be too good for her to detect. When she throws you a shit test it should glance off you like a magnet repelling the same pole on another magnet.

Shit tests from the obstacles are far less serious and easy to deflect. Just treat it like an IOD and turn your back and immediately talk to the next obstacle. If it's time to move to your target (discussed later) then so much the better, move to her. Once you are with the target, her shit test must be addressed and not ignored but as always, you never directly respond to such things.

The most famous shit test is, "I have a boyfriend." Just say, "I'm always discreet" and then move right into your next routine. Almost *never* will she be separated with you and say that and be telling the truth. It is almost always just a test and if you react in any way other than, "Great we'll party on" then you fail the test. Alpha Males don't compete, and in some ways they don't dominate... in reality, Alpha Males *just don't care!*

You probably are aware by now that you never offer a girl, and especially the target once you get to her, a compliment. Every other guy who has approached them for years has complimented them and you are Alpha Male, not "every other guy"! (Reason #20383 why Game only works on 9's and 10's.)

Some IOI's might be fakes and thinly-veiled shit tests. A girl might compliment you just to see if you fall for it. Lower-than-Alpha-Males express thanks for compliments always, or compliment back. Just to be sure it's real and not a shit test attempt, keep your compliments at a 1-to-2 ratio. Only compliment her if she's given you two. Ignore the first one, or just smile knowingly like you know what she said is true and stay on course with your routine.

An IOD can be a bored look at you talking or perhaps she will look away. You need to punish that by immediately striking up a conversation with the next female closest by. An IOD is not a sign she doesn't or won't like you. If you punish the first IOD or two, she will often improve her behavior.

For minor IODs, slip in a neg. Say this, "I like your dress [or top, whatever]; it's very popular these days." And then start the next routine. She will drop a notch after that neg and she cannot blame you because you obviously meant it as a compliment. To a female, for whatever reason, that isn't a good thing to hear no matter how unique or common what they're wearing is.

Don't Answer Questions

Early in the set, if a girl asks you something never answer! Well, never answer directly. Questions from the set are great because they are IOIs but you reward them too early if you answer their questions.

The best response to a question is, "Guess!" So if they ask how old you are, say, "Guess!" (Don't repeat their question like, "How old do you think I am?" because that shows way too much interest and attention in their question. Alpha Males don't show much attention to questions.)

Ultimately, if you really get into the set and they all fawn over you and then (as shown later) you have moved to the 10 and getting high IOIs from her, you can move into a slightly-more willing participant in answering questions. But this takes experiential practice to know when and how much and you'll get better over time.

Enthusiasm Begets Enthusiasm

Be enthusiastic at all times! You're the life of the party for the first time in your life. The reason you were not before is you had no idea what to say. I am telling you what to say and how to stand and when and where to move. You have no more excuse to be a wallflower so the option remaining is the enthusiastic life of the party. Be happy, be smiling, be calm, be comfortable, you *must* be in a don't-care attitude if you want to be in her pants.

Don't be *stupidly* enthusiastic however or you will come across as the little fraud you really are. (It's okay, you are a fraud, so was I, this doesn't come naturally; the good thing is you move from fraud to real because as you see instant results your first night out, the reinforcement of success will reinforce these skills and ingrain them in you for good.)

Try to calibrate your enthusiasm to be slightly higher and more expressional than the set's. That's it. You will wake up the set and attract them but not look freaky. Such a calibrated enthusiasm level makes you the lamppost the girls want to hover around.

Oh So Critical – Keep Your Momentum!

Right after the first opening routine, you say this to start the next one: "Listen, I've got to get back to my friends, but…" *or* say this to begin the second routine: "I only have another few seconds but…"

Such a routine opener put a *time constraint* on yourself. This serves two purposes. It shows that you have other things to do than stand around and talk to *them* all night (this is increasing your perceived value to the group and is an example of a DHV, a Demonstration of Higher Value). If you have practiced, the opposite of what you (and I) have done every other time we've been next to a woman: our value as someone they might like is increasing as the seconds go by. You are now moving up from the 7.5 or so you had risen to and if they are responding well to your opening routine you are almost certainly at the level of 8. You can drop from there fast but practice makes perfect.

And remember to keep rocking away from them, looking around. You're Alpha Male and you have lots of fish to fry.

The time constraint shows them that you have friends you have to get back to and you only have another minute or two to talk *but…* and then immediately begin your second routine. Again, it can be whichever opener from earlier you didn't use.

The 10's Early Intervention and How to Manage Her

Definitely by the time you're in the middle of your second routine the 10 is going to start feeling uncomfortably because her friends, who are not quite as hot as her, are getting your attention. Have a neg ready for when she jumps into the conversation. If it's a 3- or 4-set, you will have engaged 2 of her friends and completely not looked at her yet.

Every guy who has approached that group before you made her his focus. She is going to be desperate to get your eye by the end of your second routine.

If she says anything before that, you must neg her. Look at the two you've talked directly to (directly but indirectly too by rocking and looking around like you must be getting on your way soon) and toss the neg to them about "their friend." Make it smiley and jokey.

I gave you a couple earlier. You can ask, pointing at her smiling but immediately looking at an obstacle, such as the one you haven't yet addressed, and ask "Is she always like this? Where's her off button? [look at her just a tad] Hello, we're talking here!"

You must say this playfully with the group, not in any mean way. You are demonstrating she has lower value than she thinks and you simply are too high of value to care either way because you have a story to tell.

The following is one powerful neg and is my favorite for this situation. Look at the 10, really for the first time (you are still slightly pointed away from any one of them though) and say, "Hey, your nose sort of wiggles when you talk! No, really, it's okay. It's sort of cute." And smile and make it like you just gave her a huge compliment and then go *right back into the routine you were in.*

The nose wiggle line isn't going to be perceived by her that you were putting her down. But she will *hate* that her nose wiggles when she talks. (Obviously it may or may not wiggle, who cares? She's going to be self-conscious about it.) She will be stunned for a second. Instead of waiting with baited breath for her next platitude you just said something about her that she isn't going to like about herself. And if you're wondering what's so bad about her nose wiggling, no man can understand it but she will hate that about herself.

In many ways, you *want* the opportunity to neg her like this. You are fast-climbing to an 8.5 by interacting with her friends and she just plummeted in her mind down from the 9 she was at from you ignoring her to an 8. Read this carefully: you are now an 8.5 and she is just an 8. You just hit the jackpot baby! You're above her and she now *needs* you to want her.

Cowboy, Are You Getting It Yet?

From that previous paragraph are you seeing the dynamic that is going on here? You went from loser to someone a 10 desires in about 4 minutes! And if you practiced all this, you didn't have to think about any of it. And you are now someone she thinks is better than her and she is now going to have to *work to win you over.*

You have never in your life been in the driver's seat like this. And it's like a $500,000 Lamborghini driver's seat!

15
OTHER MEN

You aren't going anywhere there are lots of women and find no men. Great!

An advantage comes to you if a guy you know happens to pass by the set. *Always* turn and acknowledge him, shake his hand, and square right up to him. The women need to know you know that you are the Alpha Male of your friends and your friends have priority over women because you are loyal. This is known as the *leader of men* switch. When men lead, women follow.

Females constantly study your body language. Don't spend too much time with your friend. You can turn him slightly towards your set and say, "Hey girls this is Jim and we had some classes together. He's a great guy," then smile and immediately look at him, and then say to him, "Jim, I need to finish up here real fast and I'll look for you later and we'll talk." As you say the last, go ahead and turn him slightly away from the group by the arm and say, "See you in just a bit."

(I don't need to reiterate, once again, you need to practice all this do I?)

99% and almost always 100% of the men in the room have no clue about Game. The ones that do have not studied or practiced. Instead, they get a book and read the first few pages, skim the rest, never practice, and achieve tremendous mediocrity. They *do* get dates because a little Game is better than no Game. But if you take all this to heart and practice what I teach you, you will be elevated far above the other men in the room with your skillset.

If you get the resources that I demanded you get, and if you follow them in the order I gave them to you, you will be one of the few in the country who has a major foundation of skills that the pros have and only a fraction of the others who have trained under them ever achieve. Think about school and how many males actually study what they are supposed to. If you do this right, you will surpass your wildest fantasies. I am proof.

Sometimes you'll approach a set and a male will be talking to the set. He should be the first obstacle whom you befriend. You can square up to him. *Go prepared,* learn about some local or national sporting event that recently ended and learn who won, lost, and a little about perhaps one of the players. Say something to him about it, ask him if he saw the game. If he wants to get into details, say, "I don't usually follow that sport [or that team or that league depending on how much you really know] but I thought that game was awesome."

Smile at him and be enthusiastic just as you would the ladies without him. The following is critical. Ask him as you *slightly* turn to the others, "How do you all know each other?"

This is a key question. The answer tells you whether or not he is a husband, boyfriend, friend, or stranger who just walked up. Unless he's a husband or boyfriend, you're in. Once you've interacted with him and showed no interest in the females, you will have done this:

1. Disarmed him from thinking you're competition

2. Befriended him

3. Shown the women you're there for a good time, not just to meet them.

4. Shown the women you're a leader of men.

16
TIME TO ESCALATE THE ROUTINES AND THE PHYSICAL

Being the Alpha Male now, you need to be comfortable and you need to be positioned in their group as someone would be whom they accept. It's time to turn the tables somewhat on an obstacle and get into the group more physically.

If any of them are against a wall or bar facing out to the rest of the club, that is the key position you need to be in. It likely will be the 10 since she's the group's queen but it might not be. You need to be relaxed and facing out overseeing your venue that you own with the women around you. The more relaxed you are and the less that you turn to the women, the less their *protection shields* will be up and the more natural will be your entry into the set.

In addition to getting the king's position in the group, you need to be escalating your physical touch now. If you ever *have* had dates in your life, I have no doubt you were a perfect gentleman the whole time and never made a move to touch her in order to show her that you are a respectable guy she can trust. That is 90% of the reason you are a virgin.

Note: Never buy a drink for the target or obstacle. Every guy in the room will do that, let them spend their money. If anything the girls should buy you a drink. Even if you don't drink it, always accept the drink offer if anyone in the set offers it. Don't say thanks. Just say "sure" and keep talking. Don't make a big deal about it. It's their job.

Tip: The other resources explain how you can leverage your entire PUA work tremendously with a *pawn* (a female you Gamed earlier who you bring with you to the group helping to lower the set's natural protection shield) and with a *wing man*, a friend who knows what you are doing and knows how to maximize your Game in the set. (You can trade and do the same for him later or at another venue.)

It might be difficult for you at first to escalate the physical in the groups you approach but you must do this from the start, beginning with the quick arm touch in your opening routine. The 10 needs to see her friends comfortable enough to let you touch them without repelling you. And by doing it quickly and unconsciously (never look at your hand as you touch them; it's even best if you are talking to an obstacle and the moment you touch her even if it's the first-time, one-second first touch of the group look at another obstacle the moment your touch lands on the previous one and continue your routine, taking your hand off the first one a second later).

Seated Set

If the set you approach is seated in seats, as you begin your second routine right after you express the false time constraint ("I need to get back but did you know...") grab a chair and sit but do this *as you're talking*. If they are at a booth and there is room at either end, sit on the outside of the booth *as you're talking*.

Obviously there are possible problems with this. A chair might not be close. The set might be seated in a booth without any room on either end. This truly is a problem you must address... Alpha Males never stand when women are seated. Alpha Males sit with women. Alpha Males sit while women might stand. But Alpha Males never are the only ones standing.

If you cannot grab a chair or sit in the booth or couch, you perhaps should reconsider approaching that set in the first place. Wait until there is an opening or just move to a different set.

Tip: Once you get seated, always *lean back* and relax. Keep being chatty but sit back, you are enjoying the venue. Everybody is there for you. The Alpha Male enjoys the environment that is there for him. He is not there for the environment.

There are some advanced ways to steal the seat of one of them, and if you can do this for your target so much the better. It sometimes requires that you perform a combination of DHVs followed by IODs at her. The resources I strongly urged you to get and study once you finish this describe the *twirl* technique and other ways to put yourself in the best position in the group in your opening minutes.

Live the Game

It's so nice, it's worth saying about 10,000 times. You must practice all this before you try it. Unless your fragile ego can stand being blown out of the first 25 sets you try (it cannot), you should not be doing this live but in the privacy of your own bedroom. And then you practice it when you are not doing Game but just when you're going through life the next few days, ordering lunch, seeing your friends, buying comics, whatever, you Game everybody you see, yes men and women.

Alpha Males live Game. People love Alpha Males and don't know why. It's because they have Game. They smile, they speak loud enough for all their audience to hear them, they project their voices without trying, they square up to men as a loyal friend and they never really square up facing females because the whole world of females is theirs to pick from and they don't have to show interest but women have to show interest in them first.

Note: You're sometimes going to strike out. You'll go where the women are and can't even open a set. It happens. As a famous PUA named Roissy says, "Beta backsliding is a fact of life." Roissy is referring primarily to Alpha Males who once get into a relationship for long- or semi-long-term can fall out of Alpha Male mode for a while and lose the upper-hand in a relationship. But you can also fall into your beta old ways when you get blown out of sets multiple times in a night. It can be due to a number of factors and possibly *might* just be the night's make-up of women that just don't click the right way for some reason. It is often just that you are off your Game. Recalibrate. It helps tremendously to take a pocket recorder or use a smart phone app to record yourself once you notice it happening. You'll soon realize if you're honest that you are failing to show a laid-back, confident tone. Your body language might be okay but your voice isn't pulling its weight. It might also be time to recalibrate your peacocking. If you're been wearing wild T's perhaps it's time to trade those out for a more formal look. Test and try things. The Alpha Male in you will soon crawl his way to the top again.

Time for Another Routine

Once you've become a part of the group and took the leadership's physical position you will just go straight into a routine. Start it with, "Oh man, I need to get back but..."

You should know a couple of mid-Game routines. By the way, if you happen to move faster with the target due to her showing extremely signs of IOIs early, you might want to save one of these for her and the best might be the photo routine. But as long as she's still on the fringe and you've negged her once or twice then you should have prepared both of the following standard routines.

The ESP Routine

Several variations exist but the one here is the standard delivery. I would once again give credit to Mystery except I am unsure if he or Style or Matador or one of Mystery's protégées developed it.

Warning: If things are going well and the obstacles all show IOIs and the target is coming around nicely looking at you with awe or IOIs and you're in the groove and you are still calm and leaning back, you may want to escalate to the target now instead of later. In other words don't waste time doing one or two more routines with the obstacles. These pre-target routines for the whole set exist *only to build interest in the target and exist for no other reason.* I've barely mentioned the target for many pages but *she is your goal, that is why she's called the target.* So drop the routines and move to focusing on the target if you see it's already time to do so. But only experience will tell you when you can. In general, especially until you get more experience in the field, you are going to need these routines to build more attraction and build DHVs for yourself before the target is fully ripe to be plucked from the group.

Note: This all sounds like I'm really an expert, right? And too much for you to master perhaps? Nonsense. As I write this, I'm only about 10 months away from the time I had pizza with George and all this fell into my lap. I did what most guys who hear about this don't do: I got tons of materials and made this my life's work for a few months. But you don't even have to do that much work. I narrowed the resource list down from the 40 or so books, recordings, and videos I studied to the *only four that matter* for you to get and follow in that order after finishing this book. After reading this and the book *The Game*, you'll be ready to go out and open sets and begin to get practice. After Mystery's book (the second item in my resource list) you'll be fully-armed to get laid. But the honing of your skills and all the unanswered questions are fully explained in the final two resources so to be a master you need to get to the audio course ultimately. Don't skip a step. The audio course discusses topics without defining them. You need the previous resources, especially a thorough read of Mystery's book (the second resource) before the ultimate class, the audio course.

The ESP routine was made famous on *The Pick-Up Artist* TV show in your resource list. It goes like this:

"Hey, do you believe in ESP?"

It is time to begin directing your routines to the entire group at once, you're quickly becoming the group leader. So you might start the question looking at one and look to the next girl before you finish the question, then when done look at the next one. If it's a 3-set this means you will bring in the target on the final look. If it's a 2-set, the target is now about half your focus whereas before she was a non-existent part of your interest.

It doesn't matter what they respond with. As usual. They are *women* you don't need their "wisdom" on anything. So whatever they say, and don't give them much of a chance to answer either way. Again, you never really ask women anything because your attitude and body language is: I'm here to have fun and tell you things that are fun and I might ask you questions but my follow-up is far more critical than what you say. Once you've paused a fraction to get them time to process your question and begin uttering something out of their red little lips, continue with the routine as follows.

Note: Subjects such as belief and/or experiences with ESP (or exposing ESP as a fraud), famous people you know (never brag, just include your acquaintance with one of them in an interesting story that might fractionally actually be true, or not be true), a dangerous experience you've had, do they believe in ghosts, and so on are chick crack. They are pulled to such topics like graft to politicians in Chicago.

"Think of the first number that pops into your head from 1 to 4, *don't say it* just think it. Now take that number and see it in your mind on a huge billboard along the highway. Are you doing that?"

She'll utter something like, "Yes."

"Okay. On that billboard, let me think... I see the number *3!*"

She'll either be impressed or not, it doesn't matter.

You need to understand two vital things about how to deliver the ESP routine:

1. Most people respond with 3. The odds are in your favor that you will "guess" her number. To dramatically

increase your odds to something close to 90% then practice step #2.

2. Use hand motions as you deliver the ESP routine. Practice man, practice! When you say, "...into your head from 1..." then immediately with your right hand point toward her left breast and keep it there. Keep talking and say, "...to 4,.." and as you say four you point with your left hand toward her right breast. This creates a mental plumb line. (Did I mention you practice this?) Make it smooth. When the ESP routine works, it works *well*. Okay, now that you set the boundaries of the line, then when you say, "... *don't say it* just" and as you speak that, sort of jab or point with your right hand to the 3 position, about 3/4ths of the way to your left hand. Make it smooth and quick, so it's one sentence with three hand gestures. Keep it there only about a half second.

So it goes: "Think of the first number that pops into your head from 1 [your right hand points toward her left breast] to 4 [your left hand points to her right breast], *don't say it* [point/jab at the #3 position near your left hand and keep it there for about a half-second] just think it. Now take that number..." Her subconscious takes your hand position and reinforces the number three as her number.

Such routines not only build DHV but they also are *compliance tests* which show you whether or not she is and will continue to respond. The more compliance tests they follow then the more likely you'll succeed in the set.

If you guessed it, say, "I told you ESP can be powerful, let's make it more interesting.

If you guessed wrongly (which in reality means *she* chose the wrong number because you are Alpha Male), say, "See, I don't believe in ESP either but some people say if you make

ESP even more challenging that it works best. Let's test that..." and then go into this extended ESP routine:

"Picture a number between 1 [your right hand points toward her left breast] and *10* [your left hand points toward her right breast] but *don't say it* [your right hand points/jabs at the number 7 position, about 3/4ths of the way to your left hand and stays for about a half-second]. Imagine your number is the only thing on a giant billboard. Think about the billboard. Are you doing that?"

"Yes."

"On the billboard I see a... 7."

If you guessed correctly, say, "I thought you might have some ESP ability." If you guess incorrectly, say, "See, that ESP stuff either doesn't work well or you maybe don't have it. What do you think?"

And let her spout a few words and say, "Oh wait, before I leave listen, I want to show you all something..."

Note: Staying chatty and keeping women's attention requires you stack multiple routines and conversations. This means you often start one without fully finishing. You certainly never let *them* droll on and on about anything you've brought up because they will soon get bored with their vapid lack of intelligence and you will be blamed for their boredom.

Here move to the photo routine (or another routine that you grab from the resources.) The photo routine takes a little prep work once and then you can use it over and over every time you go trolling. The photo routine is great because it gets them involved with holding props and it enables you to promote a higher and higher level of DHV.

Get a set of photos, all the same size and glossiness, from your collection. If this means you have to get digital photos developed into prints do so. Go to Wal-Mart or another photo-developing place and pick up an envelope for them. If you actually have to get some developed you'll get an envelope but you want to make sure the one you take with you to the club has no date on it. Get several, the envelope you take to the club should look fairly new.

You want to select 6 to 8 pictures (no more and no less) that show you in good form of course, looking sharp but also looking Alpha and having fun. If you've been somewhere out of the country, that is by far best, if you've been with someone famous that is a close second, if you've traveled somewhere dangerous in the country such as to the mouth of an active volcano that is great too. Don't make every photo an extreme photo but you want one or two in there.

What if geeky little you happened to get a walk-on set visit with a sci-fi star in the past year or so. Or perhaps you were at a conference where someone you admire was and you got a photo. If at a movie studio, even if it was on a tour and the star happened to be walking by and you got your picture taken, say, "I was visiting the set the other day and I started talking to Sylvester Stallone there and he was telling me that if people work out more than 2 hours a *week* that the extra benefits are negligible! Can you believe it? All those people who spend an hour and a half at the gym each day are just wasting their time. And he should know."

Now, you probably don't have a picture of you and Stallone or Chuck Norris or Van Diesel or The Rock or any of those guys but the idea is this: Whoever you have picture(s) with, or wherever you've been, it should demonstrate that you are an exotic guy. You don't say you met him on a movie studio tour, you say you were talking to him the other day on the set. You don't say, "I went to Argentina seven months ago" but instead you say, "A few weeks ago in Argentina there were these girls who offered to take my picture as I was leaving the resort..."

The difference is subtle. One way you are bragging or relating a plain, boring story about yourself. The other way you are recounting an event that you, as a matter of course, were part of, as though it's nothing special. When you brag about yourself you never win. When you are downplaying in tone a story about a special person or event you were involved in it builds up yourself without *you* actually doing the building.

"Right before Hollywood came and ruined it all for two weeks, I was here on the beach at Cannes recently and..." This works obviously if you have photos of you at Cannes. Tell a story, say how these local girls were trying to get you to go swimming with them and you couldn't speak a word of it but someone finally came up who could translate. Then say, "It was kind of awkward being American and with every French girl there going topless like it was normal."

Make sure your photos match and are congruent with whatever you expand your story into.

So, you have those photos, in the envelope, in your pocket. And now that you have opened the set, completed a routine or two, developed some IOIs, hopefully negged the 10 once or twice, perhaps had to punish an IOD once from one of them, say, "Oh before I leave I want to show you these, I just got them back from the developer." Bring out your photos and begin passing them out one by one, telling the story as you go. Of the 8 pictures, perhaps only 1 or 2 show the main event and that's fine. Make the last photo in the stack some kind of good closure. Perhaps it's you on the plane or in an airport and say, "Can you believe it, right after I got on the plane after that picture was taken by my friend, the seat I was assigned to was right next to Miley Cyrus. She is much nicer than you might think she'd be." (Just pick anybody.) Talk about how much nicer she is in person than when interviewed on TV or something like that.

If they ask why you don't have a picture of the actress you were seated next to, turn it into a neg opportunity and say, "That would be sort of rude don't you think? I mean there are thousands of pictures of her, I would never impose on a nice girl like that. She appreciated that I treated her just as a nice, regular girl."

Tip: You can use your cell phone picture app but it's not as effective as the physical props of actual photos. If you have *any* picture of you with a hot girl, yes even your cousin, make sure it's in the set of photos or cell phone pictures somewhere. "Oh she's just a friend, but we enjoyed the beach that day" you will say nonchalantly if asked who she is. (This is another reason PUA skills work only on 9s and 10s. Lesser females will feel they can never compete and will reel themselves in at this point. 9's and 10's see this as a challenge and try harder to get your attraction.)

(No, I have no idea why fathers don't teach these important lessons to their sons.)

Time to Throw the 10 a Bone!

This is the perfect time to look at the 10 (not squared up physically to her though) and say something. A slight neg is a great approach for the target now, especially if you had a chance to neg her once earlier. Mystery describes a good neg for opening the target now and it is this: as you turn toward her say, "I just don't think we should get to know each other." When she asks why, you say, "You're just too much of a nice girl for me."

That neg is also called a *false disqualifier*. You disqualify yourself from her and for some reason, this makes a 10 want you more (who can understand these females?) because it takes you out of the running. She's a 10, every other guy who has spoken to her in his life either thought he could get her or was too much of a dweeb to try. You just said you couldn't have her but it's not because of a problem with *you!*

This is extremely powerful and works both as a light neg and as a false disqualifier to build attraction.

It is good to give her a prop of some kind as you begin to open up to her more and work the obstacles much less. Perhaps take off one of your chains and say "here!" and put it around her neck. Don't ask her permission, Alphas never ask permission. Just do it. As you do, say, "I want to tell you something about this, hold it for a sec." Immediately interact with the group again with a short routine, just a 3- or 4-sentence story about your baby niece and how she said your name before she said "Mommy" or "Daddy" and how precious that was to you and that her parents actually laughed and didn't seem to feel bad at all "because we are such a close-knit family."

Kino Escalation Defined

Throughout the past two routines and after the first routine's first touch on the first obstacle's arm you should move to *kino escalation* mode (from the physical energy term *kinesthetic*). Kino escalation is the practice of touching them slightly more and more each time, building rapport as a good friend would, never being overtly sexual and never touching so much that they feel freaked in any way.

A good goal would be to put your arm around one's shoulders like a "buddy" would do. You don't keep it there for long but you just do so comfortably as you are routining the set.

Warning: If you *ever* feel tension like a touch is about to be moved away from then *you must be the one to move away first.* This means remove your arm if you sense she is about to move her shoulders from your arm, this means if you ever grab one girl's (an obstacle's or eventually the target's) shoulders to turn her to you and you feel resistance, immediately stop and turn to another girl and direct your next sentence to her. Never show disappointment; why should you, *you* are the one who decided to turn from *her* she didn't turn from you. After once or twice of being punished like this, girls instinctively want your touch more. Not one of them reading this will admit it by the way. You should be well aware that the *worst person to get meeting-women advice from is from a female.*

The more success you have, and as time goes by you will have more, with the smaller touches, you eventually should escalate to the arm-around-a-shoulder for a few seconds and if you're seated then move your hand to her knee. Keep it there for 3 or 4 seconds as you talk, even if you're not talking to the one whose knee your hand is on. This may be your target's knee if you have successfully pulled her away from the group by now and is best if you do this to the target either right before or after you get her away. Do it like you didn't even notice your hand went there. Don't rub and don't squeeze. It's just where your hand happened to land for a short time while you talk.

You will gauge her willingness to be with you by that knee touch. If she keeps her knee there, then you move your hand away after about 4 seconds. If you sense she is about to move her knee away (you *can* sense this), as before *you move first*. This takes the power from the woman and just keeps giving it to you more and more. It's like a shit test she throws you that you never fail, she loses by doing throwing out the test.

Why Nice Guys Finish Last

One primary reason you've never progressed past the "let's be friends" stage or, "You're like my brother!" stage – if you ever got *that* far with a female (I never did) – is because you didn't escalate the kino soon enough. If you wait too long to show a 100% comfortable touching comfort then you'll never get physical.

Kino escalation improves *comfort building*. The set feels more and more comfortable with your touch the more you do it but you must begin with small, almost unconscious touches that makes them think you're just a normally touchy guy and not offensive and not aggressive. Once you're with the target this is critical to move the target to enough comfort building that they are willing to bounce to another venue with you that night, if that is your plan. Or if you just are trying to *number close*, meaning get a phone number, the more comfort you build, especially by kino escalation, the better your chances are at getting a real phone number.

Nice guys wait up to three dates to begin kino. By then they are just a nice guy, never a guy the girl feels comfortable enough to have physical attraction to. The PUA knows that the earlier kino escalation begins, the far faster the female will be comfortable with contact *of all kinds*.

17
JUST YOU AND THE TARGET – YOUR FIRST 10 AND SHE'S WITH YOU AFTER ONLY 8-12 MINUTES OF TALKING!

You must now begin moving to the target. She is wet wanting to know you better (maybe not completely sexually wet (but maybe) but certainly wet with giddiness wanting more attention that she was always used to getting before you – You're now this mysterious, chatty, confident, Alpha Man who came into her picture). She is beginning to hate her friends because they have your attention. If you have done everything well to this point, the rest is actually extremely simple: Moving her away from the group so you can begin working her one-on-one.

Trust Me, I Was You... I Am Still You in All Ways Except for the Females

I would never steer you wrong. You bought my book and you will not trust me if I don't discuss all my own failures (as

I've done – the first half of this book was a picture of a total loser idiot – me) and I must be honest with my successes as well as yours. When you first learn of this stuff you are going to be intimidated but also excited, right? You are right now. You are thinking, "I have tools I never knew existed!" That is absolutely true.

You have to understand that the odds are, the first few times out you *probably* will not get to this point where you can separate the target from the group. You will *perhaps* be blown out of the group by them getting distracted or just losing interest in you the first few times out. Great! You are getting some failures out of the way and learning where you are weak and where you need to practice.

Hot women often are rude to nice guys and guys they lose interest in fast. If you begin to let a conversation drag, it means you are not projecting and your stories or photos have too much detail and not enough interest-building subjects. You learn every time you fail and you will see that when you adjust you get further and further as you learn where you get blown out of the set. Don't be offended if she says something rude like, "I have better things to do" and walks off. This is a 10's protection mechanism and it doesn't mean she is normally bitchy to everybody. She simply cannot spend time listening to every guy who talks to her and she's learned from losers before you that sometimes they don't take "no" easily so they up the exit ante and say something direct and leave.

One problem I had at first was getting everything in the proper sequence. George is awful at teaching. The books, TV shows on PUA, and the audio course has to be sequential. I have to write this one page after another and one chapter after another. Yet, much of this happens at the same time. You just learned about kino escalation in the previous chapter but you must be doing it from the set's opening routine.

So at this point it seems difficult but certainly worth doing, right? It turns out not too difficult but it's just new to you right now. So relax. And know that failure when you go out the first few times shows you exactly where your routines need work.

And so what do you do once you work on the rough places? You go back out the next night and get further. Yes, you do the very same thing; you open the sets the same way, your routines are the same, and so on.

Moving to the 10

At this point, you've addressed the target perhaps by giving her a prop like a chain and you told her you'll get back to that and now is the time. Look at her and say, "Your nails look nice, are they fake? Really, well, they still look good." Be sincere and do not *ever* say this like it's a bad thing. (She won't like it but she will blame herself and not you.)

Say, "Hey I want to tell you something" and stand and put out your arm, elbow toward her, like you are waiting for her to put her arm in yours. One of two things will happen:

1. If you were successful at everything before, you have high DHVs, you have lots of IOIs, you are the lifeblood of the set, and all the girls enjoy and trust you and you've touched them all by now. The target will almost certainly trust you enough to follow your lead and put her arm in yours and stand to begin following you. As you put your arm out, say to the obstacles, "Hey guys, do you mind if I borrow her for a minute?" but don't wait for an answer, just keep moving like they are saying "Sure, just come back soon and talk to us some more!" You should have plenty of group trust by now that they will never mind you taking the target. Plus, they feel good about your interaction and about themselves now thanks to you and you are taking away their primary competition for a while! If all goes like

this *and it will as you perfect the preliminary materials in the previous pages* then you just scored time alone with a 10 in eight to twelve minutes!

2. If you were not fully successful at the preliminaries you will sense a hesitation. If you do, pull your arm away (never let her show you resistance first) and say, "Oh by the way guys, did you know that..." and do another short routine. Try to offer a small neg along the way to the target too (it's vital to knock her down a peg without her knowing why she feels knocked). Have a routine ready that builds more demonstrations of higher value without you bragging, such as when you had to save your little sister when your house caught on fire and the fire department sirens were way too far off to wait any longer and it was just you and your mom outside. Don't brag, say something like, "You know, I didn't even feel the burning smoke in my lungs until long after I got her out of that bedroom and into the night air. It's true that when family is in danger, instincts kick in immediately." Be kino escalating the whole time, touching all of them but never long enough to be weird. Once you have a good vibe, offer another time constraint such as, "Oh man, I have to get back to my friends, they're going to be upset I've been gone so long. By the way, and immediately go back to #1 above and offer your arm once more and follow #1 verbatim. (#1 should never fail a second time. If it does, you *might* want to move to another set. Just do so while on top, meaning before the target verbally or physically is able to demonstrate she isn't taking your arm just because you offered.)

So you now are bumping the target to a more secure place in the club. As she is next to you and you begin walking, tell her, "It's so hard to say what I wanted to get your opinion on with everything going on back there." (The truth is *you* were the one going on.) (You chatty Cathy!)

Move her to a wall or better a table or best a couch (if the club has such an area) or a glass-enclosed area perhaps for pool players or somewhere the music isn't as loud and the environment is slightly more intimidate. In some clubs there isn't such a place or if there is, it's too crowded. If so, never show disappointment, just find a corner or a place by a wall as far away from "crowd" as you can and go right into the next routine. As you walk, just keep moving ahead, you're the leader she is the follower of you, the Alpha Male.

Note: If you can grow up pretending to be Luke Skywalker, you can pretend to be an Alpha Male.

The routines you do with her alone will be more intimate and your negs should be less. Actually, unless she gives you IODs you don't neg her again. You never want to punish good behavior. You will actually begin to reward her, not with typical compliments but with your own IOIs and compliments, always 2-for-1. If she's smiling and responding you can give her about half that interest back. As you develop more and more rapport there separated from the group you can increase the proportion of your IOIs to hers but never *ever* overdo them. She needs to realize that a pearl of great price is not for the asking.

The Prop

If she has a prop of yours, and she might depending on how you handled the pre-move routines, then you have to have a short story about the chain or hat or special picture or coin or whatever prop it was that you used to lock her in. Once you are more secluded with her, get that over with. Perhaps it's a coin you carry that was the only thing in your pocket when you won a sharpshooting championship or when you came in first in a talent show where you did something special.

At this point you want to begin focusing on her in ways that nobody else does. Just get the excuse routine for getting her aside over with quickly without giving her a chance to ask many questions and start the next routine.

Questions are now good although they won't be typical questions like, "Where do you work?"

When she asks you questions like that, don't respond directly but say, "What do you think someone like me would do?"

If you work in a video rental store, you want to talk about how to you in the film business doing some distribution work for a national company. If you work at a sporting goods store you are a sports distributor for athletes. Get it? You don't have to lie but you often have to improvise.

But many of you are just students! You should definitely be a student "working a marine biologist career." If you are only a student but you've written comic book story with you and your two fanboy buddies, then you are "just a student biding my time until I can complete my four novels in this series I am writing. I would love to get your take on them sometime if you'd be willing to read them."

If you haven't much to say to her question, or even if you do, you still don't want to give a lot of details. And throwing it back onto her with, "What do you think a guy like me would be interested in?" (women love guessing games like that) or asking her to sometime tell you what she thinks or your novels/paintings/furniture restoration or whatever you've sort-of-kind-of done at some point, it deflects you are just a student or a part-time retail clerk somewhere. Then you continue with the more personal routines and IOI trading, always kino escalating.

You are only minutes away from the kiss. Don't leave me yet, I am not lying to you.

Personal Routines

At this point, things get far easier even though you will right now feel far more pressure because it's just you and she. But all of the hard work is done. You don't have to have as many routines or canned material. You can begin to improvise. But you may not be good at improv until you've been in this position a few times and gotten a feel for what works for you and what doesn't.

Yes, if she gets bored the first few times and wants to get back to the group, or worse, goes to the bathroom and when done she's back with the group and not you, forget her. Actually when she does leave you for the bathroom you need to be opening another group close to where you and she were just in case. When she comes back or when she looks over after ditching you, she will regret it if she sees you have moved to someone else without thinking twice about her. About 50% of the time she will come back to you. You then can use her as instant DHV to the new group, meaning they will see this 10 showing you interest and you then can decide to go after the new group's 10 or moving back with the other one you've invested time with. Obviously you can't overlap routines when she comes to the new group so don't repeat the same ones if she's in earshot. But her return is a major IOI and her ditching you may have just been a shit test you passed far better than she ever thought you would because you ignored her leaving and got another group before she had a chance to empty a cupful of pee from her bladder.

So I'd suggest at first, leave the new set by saying, "Oh, hey guys I've got to get back to our conversation but we'll meet up later!" and take the target back to the seclusion.

The routines need to be personal now.

A good one is this famous question: "I see you have a lot of going for you, but lots of women are good-looking and looks fade. What besides just looks are attractive qualities about you?"

Unless she has previously been worked by a PUA she has *never* been asked this before. She will have to think for a minute. As she talks, if something she says triggers a quick story that might build DHV, segue to it and then return. You want to keep stacking stories, swapping back and forth threads you and she began.

Once you finish that, ask this: "So I'm just trying to see what's really underneath. If you could be anyone in the world, what would be your dream?" then *quickly add,* "and don't say princess!"

She will also have problems with this question. She is feeling now that she really isn't worthy of you at all. You are in the driver's seat! Never show disappointment no matter how lame her answers are but never show any extreme interest either. Just a casual interest. You want to show her more interest and look into her eyes more than you did the group's obstacles that's for sure. She needs to be rewarded for being there with you and showing you IOIs. But you still are the Alpha Male. It takes a lot to impress you but she's beginning to get more of your attention.

Physical Routine Time

You need a physical routine. Do you believe in the power of palm reading? Yeah, nobody in his right mind does. But that shouldn't stop you from reading her palm and blowing her away with your ability.

Subjects such as palm reading and ESP are such that even Christian girls who know that stuff is nothing more than just New Age crap get hooked into wanting to see what you're going to do.

Note: About Christians... If you are a Christian and you are thinking you won't sleep with her before marriage – well, that's even better. You will *want and need this Game material to get married.* I think you're better for it to be happy with one woman. Studies *always* show married people live longer, make more money, and are happier than two people who aren't married. You won't sleep with her before marriage? Great, you have some time to build and incredible attraction that will be a bond forever, a bond that neither time not minor problems after marriage can ever break. The attitude here about Alpha Male and women who want to follow is simply using *their personalities for you to get to know one of them better.* All you've heard from your church friends about "being yourself and being nice" hasn't gotten you anywhere. As a matter of fact, the Godly men of Scripture were bold and all were Alpha Males while at the same time they always demanded respect *for* women and you should always respect them too if you want to be like those men were. It was the girly men like Judas and Caiaphas who were the losers. The Pontius Pilate guys who were in leadership positions but couldn't make up their minds about the most obvious of things were the enemies, never the heroes. None of this Game material is disrespecting women. It is simply utilizing their innate personalities to make you the man they are attracted to. You are changing *yourself* not them. The difference between Alpha Males and betas (aka, losers) is not the women, it's the men and the way the men behave. You aren't forcing women to do anything. Why shouldn't Christian men all have happy and beautiful 10s as wives and let the heathens have nothing but ugly, bitchy chicks who wear the pants in the relationships, make all the rules, and sleep around on their weak, limp-wristed, skirt-wearing husbands?

Palm reading routines work a lot like the ESP routine you saw earlier. They play on odds and emotion to impress their targets. You can become a master at it simply by googling "palm reading" and you'll see it's just another way to use someone's built-in emotional makeup to flip attraction switches for you.

On one of the more popular PUA boards (http://www.pick-up-artist-forum.com), a user named Handsome Artist took from several sources and put together his own palm reading system for when he wants to *close* a girl. By closing, it can mean you will "close" the sale to get her number, kiss her, bounce her to another location, or any number of things which means taking the meeting with her to a higher level. The reason palm reading is so popular is because it works well. It's not something to discount just because it sounds silly; it is silly. But it works.

Palm reading escalates kino because you have her hand in hers. This is great because during the reading you'll be holding her hand in one of yours and drawing your fingers across the top of her palm with your other hand. This increases the feeling of intimacy and it also raises her sense of you being her authority and her following you.

Note: Being able to take her hand and hold it long enough to perform a palm reading is exactly why you have been escalating the kino throughout, first with the obstacles and then with her as you handed her a lock-in prop, perhaps touched her a few times as you were getting her ready to bounce to this secluded location, and then offered your arm, elbow bent toward her, to put her arm in yours and follow you. All of that lesser kino was *comfort building* for her, showing her that touching you never ended with any problem and actually was always rewarded with a cool fun and chatty conversation (routine) with you.

Throughout the whole palm routine, keep it light and smile. Don't laugh at yourself doing it but just remain friendly and happy and never take the routine seriously. Of course, you never take any of these routines seriously. Still, it's like you want to show her something she'll want to know about.

Here is Handsome Artist's take, with a few minor edits on my part to make it flow better here:

This routine is set up to be a closer, but it's up to you where to take it. You use it once you've isolated or bounced your target and you are trying to build comfort and emotional investment. The hand contact is great kino.

Once you are isolated put your hand out and say "give me your hand. Some say that I can sense a person's life force or energy level from their palm or by the mere touch of their hand, although maybe I'm just a great sensor of people." (This is good time for a "fake nail neg.") [When you see her hand, ask, "Oh, are your nails fake?" Whatever she says, say, "Oh... well they are nice,"]

Keep it just flirting and entertaining. Keep the reading light and playful. Tell her lots of positive things about herself. [This is a rewarding routine for her, one that should increase her comfort with you and her enjoyment that she accompanied you to the secluded place.]

Here is a link to a diagram showing the lines used in palm reading. Get familiar with them, but they don't really matter that much because she shouldn't be looking at her hand, you should be making good eye contact with her while you talk to her.

(http://www.divineanswers.com/wp-content/uploads/2008/11/palm-reading-marriage-line.jpg)

First, make general flattering assertions about her. For example, pick out a few of these:

• You're Hard-working and dependable

• You're Friendly

• You're Kind and considerate

• You're Loyal and honest

• You're a Problem solver

- *You're Good at completing tasks*

- *You're Fun to be around*

- *You're Flexible and adaptable*

- *You're Bright and capable*

- *You're a Natural leader*

- *You're Independent and resourceful*

- *You're Cooperative and friendly*

- *You're Good-natured*

- *You're a Good communicator*

- *You're Family-minded*

- *You have excellent people skills*

  Now tell her some things about her life such as:

- *You do not like to compromise your principles.*

- *I sense that you are more entrepreneurial, than domestic.*

- *The success in your career has not always been reflected in your personal life.*

- *You sometimes have dreams of flying, which means you have a very strong spirit – you are not going to be confined by life's limitations.*

- *Also tell her you feel strong energy from her which may indicate that she possesses some kind of psychic or intuitive ability. Legitimize this by asking her if she ever has deja vu, or knows the phone is going to ring before it does.*

- *Also tell her she has an old soul, and relate her to someone famous from a past era like roman, Egyptian etc...*

Now talk about her love life:

- *Sometimes you attract the wrong type of man.*

- *Older men are often attracted to you, though you are looking for a certain type of man and most of those do not fit the bill.*

- *If you date a man, more than three times, it has the potential of being a serious relationship.*

- *You have no tolerance for men who are jealous or lack confidence.*

Now if you're getting good IOI's at this point you can get deeper and suggest that you two are made for each other. (This gets her panties wet!)

Say some things like:

- *Finding your soul mate is important to you.*

- *My impression is that there is a long-term relationship in your past that did not work out. I see this man as someone who has tried to stay in your life by becoming your friend, rather than a romantic interest. I sense you want more than he has to offer.*

- *When you meet the person of your dreams, you will know it at once. You will feel the chemistry between you. He will be taller than you with an unmistakable sparkle in his eyes. I see some significance with the initials – (whatever your initials are)*

At this point your voice should be low and intense. making strong eye contact, and practically noses to nose (I suggest breath mints) and drop the hammer and kiss close.

The Kiss Close

It's time to kiss her. Right then and there. Might be the first kiss of a girl in your life actually be a 10? Why not start at the top and then just stay there? Men who start with 5's and think they will work themselves up higher on the rating ladder never do.

The *kiss close* is a routine that ends in you kissing her. A lot of guys know several kiss closes but in the end, they go back to using the standard one that works best: The famous Mystery kiss close.

Yes, sport, it's time to do it. You just met a beautiful woman, one you would never have spoken to before reading this book. And after meeting her 20-30 minutes ago you're about to swap saliva. Scary huh? It was for me too, except I was just following the program George taught me. I can be a programmed robot for love! You can too.

And the move to kiss her is *so easy* even we geeks can do it.

Here it is:

You'll be looking into her eyes after the palm reading routine. You look right at her, face to face, and ask, "Were you wanting to kiss me?"

If she does not lean to you immediately and kiss you, she will say one of three things:

1. "Yes," and you do so immediately.

2. "Maybe" (or anything like that such as, "I don't know" or "Well...") then you say, "Let's find out" and you kiss her immediately.

3. "No," where you say, "I didn't say you *could* kiss me, it just looked as though you had something on your mind.

If she answers "no" and you mess up by asking her "why not?" then you have just blown yourself out for the night by showing you're not Alpha. Alpha's don't care. That awful response showed a complete inability to be disqualified by her.

A "no" will be extremely rare if you've done everything correctly until that point. As a matter of fact, if you sensed any hesitation during the palm reading routine where you thought she might be uncomfortable with you holding her hand so long, you could finish that routine and instead of moving to the kiss close, you could keep talking by starting another routine. This is why you practice and have a couple of back-up routines memorized. Anything that indirectly shows something heroic you did, or something you did to help your baby sister or little cousin is great to build comfort and to build your DHVs.

If she does deny you the kiss close, you are still in the Game due to your Alpha response of, "I didn't say you *could* but it looked as though you had something on your mind." So you go right into another routine and keep doing kino escalation. She might offer to kiss you if you are on your Game well and not taken down a notch by her rejection. It may not have been hesitation on her part but one final shit test that you passed with flying colors. So don't get down over the "No" which again will be rare. If she doesn't kiss you first, after another routine or two and kino escalation that she doesn't seem to shy away from, you should probably go for the number close to get her number for a call later in the week (see below). If you number close then after another routine, take her hand (never yank it but never ask for it, Alphas just take), look at her in the eyes, look at her lips, look at her in the eyes, and if she is following your lead then kiss her. If you sense *any* hesitation from her then say, "Hey, I really do need to get back to my buddies but it's been interesting." (Don't thank her or say how wonderful it's been talking to her! You were doing *her* the favor, an Alpha never thanks women for doing them the favor of being in his presence.) If you think the kiss is possible after another routine or two and she follows your lead on looking into your eyes, then lips, then eyes, just lean in and kiss her.

All this discussion of what to do after a "No" is simply fire insurance. Most of the time you get the kiss close and it's Game on. When you kiss her, either thanks to the kiss close or later at some point, put your hand on the back of her neck and sort of pull her head even more to you. Don't put pressure on her neck, just show you're in charge. Women often melt at this because they finally have a man who knows them, who understands them (even though you don't, none of us ever do), and who is taking care of their emotional needs.

Warning: When you succeed at the kiss close, you are not in the end Game! *You* should stop the kissing after a few minutes. Leave her wanting more, you're Alpha Male and can kiss anytime you want so you have the freedom to cut it off and do something else. The next chapter is the "something else."

A parting thought about the kiss close. It is possible that there is a technical reason why she will not kiss you. Her friends might be within eyesight or she thinks she has bad breath and doesn't want to offend you. Although the three kiss close options are definitely the most common responses, if she says, "Not right here" or "Yeah, but not right now," then that's a good sign she wants to and ultimately will do so. Your response should be simply, "I understand," pull back a little from her face, and then start the next routine before number closing and possibly bouncing to a different venue.

18
THE END GAME

You have the girl. You've pulled her aside, you've done one or more routines, you might even have done some improv with conversation giving her some IOIs in return for more IOIs from her. It's time to answer the question, "What's next, sport?"

Obviously you want to sit there and keep kissing her but the problem with that is that either she will want to keep kissing or she will soon want to stop. If she wants to keep kissing and gets passionate and wants more physical from you right then, are you ready for it? Do you have a place if that is what you're going for? You don't want to say, "Well, my car is outside, we can go there since my Mom is home..."

Tip: If you bounce her to a different location and when you two get in your car if she starts tearing your clothes off you, obviously your car is a fine place to move things up a notch. But it's never *your* choice if your goal is to get sex because it shows desperation. Even Alphas know to take her to a hotel or to his apartment for sex unless she makes it clear she will do it in the club bathroom or in your car or someplace like that.

It's sort of difficult to know what to do after you successfully kiss close and you have to develop a sense for it fast. But you certainly should attempt to cement things better with a bounce to a different venue. She is feeling comfort, and by you being the one who (temporarily) ended the great kissing, she has more affirmation that you are not just a guy who *only* wants her for her body (even if you do).

If you go for a number close right now, it might be putting a damper on a night together that she might not be ready to end just yet. The best way to gauge is to bounce her to a different venue. If it's walkable, such as a coffee shop down the street, so much the better. She won't have to worry about being in your car alone with you and get nervous. But she has been kissing you in public and she only met you 20-30 minutes ago so she definitely has some trust going with you. So if a car is the only option for the bounce, you'll be offering it.

Note: Remember, every bounce feels like a different date to her. This greatly fast-forwards the time factor between meeting and getting her in the sack or into a more traditional relationship.

The Bounce

Keep your tone light and friendly. Say, "Hey, all of my friends might be going to another club a little later but for now why don't we go grab a coffee with me at Starbucks across the street?" It could be a slice of pizza or just a drink in a more private nearby bar that isn't seedy.

Notice you don't ask her. But you also don't just take her by the hand and lead her out of the club for the bounce. There are too many factors not in your control. She might be the driver for her friends for example although a 10 is rarely the one driving. She might want to check in with her friends before leaving just to get their tone before leaving with you. If so, go with her and be buddies with all of them and say, "We hope you didn't get too bored without us!" when you get back to them.

The dynamic has changed though and you and she are beginning to be an item and she doesn't want to look slutty to her friends for leaving with you. You can take the reigns and say, "Tina and I were thinking about going to get a coffee for a few minutes across the street. Can you girls keep this place going until we get back?"

Probably the bounce will happen. And if it's coffee or perhaps pie and coffee, yes, it's probably something you should pay for even though you're Alpha. Hey, she's a 10 who kissed you. If that doesn't deserve pie, I don't know what does.

If you can then bounce to yet another place, such as a different club after a quick coffee, so much the better because that certainly means a car ride with you and more comfort building. The whole way you are still the guy with the smile who just loves life. Talk about your recent trip somewhere. Now here is where you must be careful though if you don't have a place for sex. You might be closer to sex than you realize. So you either fish or cut bait.

If you absolutely don't have a place ready then you'd better have one next time, or else you'd better be able to say you're saving yourself for a special girl and you want to find out if she is that special girl with another date, perhaps a daytime date. This buys you time and if you do want to delay sex until you have a place for it or even until marriage (I'm surprised you originally bought this book given its title if you're looking sole for wife material, but I am thrilled because it's going to find you your lifelong partner much faster than you ever thought possible) then you two will become date mates for a while to see how things work. In the meantime, you still should be clubbing to keep all options open. You don't know this girl and they always turn out somewhat differently from our first experiences with them.

The Number Close

For whatever reason the bounce just doesn't always work or you just won't be ready for it. (Shame on you for not having enough confidence in your skills to have planned for it ahead of time.) If so, say, "I need to be going but [hand her your cell phone] here, put your cell phone number in my phone."

Never ask for her number. Just assume it's coming and by putting it into your phone it saves you the awkward moment of trying to find something to write with. Besides, Alphas never dictate, only women take dictation...

If she asks when you will call, smile big and say, "Soon!"

When she hands your phone back, don't make any promises but do say, "It was interesting being with you for several reasons actually. [Don't be bothered to list them. Always be coy and keep her guessing.] It is nice to find a girl who isn't wrapped up in her looks." She will have no idea if this is a good thing or a bad thing.

When do you call her? You probably know my answer, certainly you wait at least two or three days. If you call and get her voice mail, leave a quick message telling her to call you back. Then do *not* call again for three days. If she has not called you back, call her one more time. If she answers mention nothing about her not returning your call. Say, "I've been really busy or I might have called sooner. Why don't you meet me at [bar or coffee shop] Friday at 6:00?" Keep the call short and make a date. If she hesitates, be cool and don't even act as though you notice. Tell her you need to get off the phone because a friend is coming over to cook you dinner tonight and you have to get dressed and then wish her a good night. At that point, don't call back unless she calls you first; she has your number from your call to her cell.

(A friend who comes over and cooks you dinner, by the way, is *never* a guy and she knows it. This increases her sense of loss and improves your chance she will call you back.)

Now all of this is to handle the possibility that she won't want to see you again. You must be ready to handle that correctly because nobody has trouble handling a woman who wants him and who says "Yes" to all his suggestions. The odds are good she will want to see you again. The techniques above give you a blueprint of how to go about moving her forward again if she seems to be having second thoughts. And she's only a 10 in an ocean of 10's. If you feel *any* rejection you need to cure it by going out after the phone call and working some sets using the 3-second rule. You'll forget about her and get another. By the time you do that, the first one will probably be calling and you just pick and choose as an Alpha Male would do.

19
WHAT NOW?

Do you have more questions than answers?

That isn't entirely true and you should be honest here. If this is your first time learning about this stuff, your jaw is probably still dropping from the realization you gleamed throughout the past several chapters that this stuff *might just work!*

Only there is no *might* about it. These are powerful techniques that use the woman's nature to view *you* as the man she wants. You are simply pushing the buttons she is giving you. If 10s reacted differently, this book would be different. But the fact is that 10s react to leaders by following them. 10s react to negs by wanting the guy even more who's negging her. Once you begin showing her interest, especially as you bump her to a more secluded spot in the club after basically ignoring and negging her for a few minutes beforehand, she will actually believe that *she* was successful in *getting your attention* when it was exactly the opposite.

And she never has to know you were a loser geek. Never admit it. Just be the cool guy you now know how to be: laid back, always friendly, loving the world, leader of men, and a guy women follow. You don't have to be physically big to be a leader of men. (Think Napoleon Bonaparte.) You lead men in ways similar to women except they are already in your club if they are friendly and good-looking guys and jocks. In other words, you always square up to them, talk clearly and loudly enough so they hear you the first time, shake hands, introduce yourself (have you noticed you *never* introduce yourself to women? Don't be the dunce that most guys are, an introduction is the worst way to break into a set), even possibly buy the guy a drink if you hit it off a couple of minutes. That's all there is to leading men and women follow not only leaders of women but leaders of men.

Never buy women drinks; rules are made to be broken but *never* buy them drinks when you first meet them for sure. They should buy them for you if anything – if they ask during your first 20-30 minutes, "How about a drink?" always answer with a big smile, "Sure, thanks!" and make sure you're working a set near you when she returns with your drink. Even if you aren't consuming alcohol, tell her you'll have whatever she's having and then nurse it as long as you're with her. Or possibly just set it down after a few moments and forget about it. This shows her you can't be bribed and she has to work harder for you.

If you're working a new set when she leaves to get you a drink – and if you're not, what's wrong with you? – then introduce her to your new friends, not by name but say how you're telling them about such and such (don't tell her you just met them) and decide if you use her to increase your chances at someone in the new set or just use the set to demonstrate higher value to her.

The Resources Are Your Next Step

Yes, I'm about to go into a little detail about Comic-Con, but honestly at this point that is sort of boring. Boring to you, not to me; I remember ever little detail, down to the last touch, smell, and taste!

Your job now is to go back through this book and re-read it more slowly this time. Now that you understand the philosophy of it all, reading about Game from the start and reviewing opening the set through the kiss close and bounce or number close will sink in far more.

And it's time for you to get the resources without hesitation. Especially the two books so you can fill in the answers on the questions I may not have answered. You'll be going out long before you get to the third resource, the TV show episodes that you must watch, because the first two resources will reinforce what I've taught you here and will give you a few more details, especially the second one that is more like a textbook than a novel or description.

By the time you begin the audio sets at the end of the resources you should be well into meeting girls and kiss closing if nothing else. The audio course works like a Master's Thesis though, pulling everything you have learned from me and will learn from the others (especially Mystery since the resources are Mystery-material-heavy and he is the original master and creator of so many proved techniques), that once you're into those audios you will be in the top 1% of the top 1% of PUAs. Keep in mind, most guys won't get past Strauss's book *The Game*, the first resource to get, before they think they know enough and will stop learning. They will get women but not nearly as often as you if you trust me and get and read, watch, and listen to every one of the resources.

20

A FUNNY THING HAPPENED AT COMIC-CON

I entered a virgin and left smelling like a rose.

Literally.

Her name actually *was* Rose.

What Happened

I did attend Comic-Con planning to get laid. It was not actually something I had built myself up to expect because I didn't want to be disappointed. Plus, at fanboy conventions the 3's outnumber the 10's by factors of 20 or more. Still, Comic-Con is different with lots of industries and representatives and attendees who do not normally go to other similar conventions so I knew there would be enough supply to have a shot. And I knew there would be so many geeks dressed as Spock that I would stand out like a knight riding a white horse when I walked into that conference dressed in my navy blue, 100% all natural fiber suit, with button-down collar and silk regimental stripped tie.

Note: I am *so* grateful for our casual society. Used to, all men wore suits. Now it's rare and even more rare at conferences and *most* rare at comic book conferences. I have peacocked clubs before in some loud shirts and hats and all that. But it's nice to peacock in the opposite way, being the only one dressed like an Alpha Male is supposed to feel.

Anyway, I overspent and got a room at the Hard Rock San Diego hotel just one block from Comic-Con. I had to pay far more for it than the hotels three to seven miles away where most others stayed but I had my sights on my possible tryst so I needed to be prepared. And I had developed a high skill set back home in the months after George introduced me to Game at Carlos's Pies in December.

I upgraded my Hard Rock Hotel room to a mini-suite. It was slightly larger than a deluxe room and since I wasn't sharing a room with George as we'd done the year before (he had his own similar plans for Comic-Con too and although we drove there together he was staying further away). The mini-suite felt large since it would just be me staying there.

George and I got to San Diego and checked in the afternoon before Comic-Con began. He kept the car because his hotel was farther away (even though we had driven my Civic there). Before I left my room next morning, the first day of Comic-Con, I put my clothes away and my toiletries back in my suitcase. I did this because Alpha Males are neat and tidy by design (if not by nature).

My plan was this: No matter whether she was working at the conference as part of the wait staff, clean-up crew, vendor booth, or an attendee like me, if I saw a 10 I would Game her. I'd go up and over-the-shoulder tell her about a girl fight I just saw or tell her a funny story. I saw four 10's in the first 30 minutes and was a little disappointed because I thought I would have seen more by then. On two of them I used the Elvis opener:

"Hey, did you know that Elvis died... [the briefest of pauses]... his hair?"

Obviously you took that to a different place than it first starts to sound.

"Yeah, it's the craziest thing, do you know what his natural hair color was?"

"No what?"

"Guess." [Rarely answer questions girls ask when you first approach them.]

No matter what they spout out, say, "Dirty blonde! I couldn't believe it when I learned that. There is no way Elvis would have made it big if he hadn't, early on, dyed his hair jet-black. Can you imagine a dirty-blonde Elvis singing 'Love Me Tender, Love Me True'?!"

One of the girls immediately was approached by someone in the booth she was working. I think it was her boss because he told her to handle some sign problem and she looked at me sort of with puppy dog eyes and said, "I've got to go." I think she expected me to wait or do more, perhaps leave my number, so I said, "Great me too" and I turned and left.

I did plan to return later but never got back there. The other one I pulled the Elvis opener on laughed and talked for bit. She was an attendee but was with a mixed group of co-workers and they all seemed to have sort of a game plan for the conference and she just didn't do much with the bait I sent her way with the Elvis opener so I just turned and continued walking.

I was not down at all. It was only my first morning there.

Then I spotted a booth about four more booths down with what looked to be two hotties without anyone showing any interest in their booth.

Thanks to the *The Pick-Up Artist* TV show (in your resource list) I was able to pull this one off beautifully on that 2-set. Both were 10s working a booth for some unknown film animation company and nobody was at their booth. It was lame and the girls were bored, a perfect opportunity for Game.

I walked by and acted as though I hadn't seen them. I could feel their eyes on me. Remember, I was dressed to the nines as they say, far better dressed than anybody else who had passed them that day and I was smiling and carefree. Plus it was early and they were probably thinking if they were already bored, what were they going to be like by the show's end?

When I passed right in front of them, I sort of acted as though I spotted them out of the corner of my eye and said this:

"Hey, I was listening to a morning talk show in my suite this morning before I left for the convention. I couldn't believe they were talking about women taking baths, did either of you hear it?"

They nodded their heads "No," back and forth like those bobble dogs you see in the back windows of cars.

"It turns out that studies show that 92% of all females masturbate in the bathtub!"

[Pause just a moment...]

"And do you know what the other 8% do?"

Again, as expected, they nodded their heads "No," back and forth like those bobble dogs you see in the back windows of cars. Only this time they had a little glint in their eyes because I hooked their interest with that opener.

"They sing" I exclaimed!

[Pause for only half a moment...]

"And do you know *exactly* what they supposedly sing?"

"No, what?" they said almost in giddy unison.

[Pause... turning slightly at them then looking back around as though I am talking not just to them but confiding what I just learned to an imaginary friend...] "You don't know what they sing? Well... I guess we know what *you* do in the bathtub!"

After a brief pause – it takes women a little more time to get obvious jokes like that than men – they both burst out laughing, looked at each other, then both looked at me laughing still, and one began twirling a little bit of hair (an IOI, and this is extremely early for an IOI but I was used to the signs by now) and I sort of sauntered over and said, "You know, I have to get back to my friends over on the next aisle soon but did you know..."

And the Game was on.

It turns out they just finished their freshmen year at some San Diego college and they had been roommates there. (I saw no reason to tell them I had just graduated high school.) We bantered about some and it turns out their names were Chrissy and Rose and both were stunning. Chrissy was a blonde with long golden hair and a low-cut blouse. Rose was more conservatively dressed but had the cutest button nose I'd ever seen. I prefer brunettes like Rose over Chrissy but I'm nothing if not open-minded and I'd be happy with either being the target. I was sort of at a loss as to how to proceed since this was a 2-set consisting of only two targets.

I wasn't sure which to cozy up to and which to neg but the decision was made for me fast when Chrissy got a cell phone call and said, "It's Tim, I need to take this, he's my boyfriend working the LucasArts booth on the other side this building" and off she went to talk to him in private.

Rose was then all of a sudden alone with me, and it has never happened before, but has since, that we basically went from opener to seclusion instantly. She showed lots of IOIs and wouldn't break her eye contact with me. I sort of kept my side toward her and kept people-watching as we spoke because I needed to maintain proper body language to make this work. If I showed weakness, I'd break the spell. I could *not* show the interest I was feeling.

But I negged her only once and it wasn't even a real neg. Never fall into patterns, each set is different. If she shows IOIs early and you sense nothing else you don't neg her because she should never be punished for acting great towards you. At some point, I asked the usual question, "So lots of girls have their looks but beauty fades. What more do you have going for you?"

After about 6 minutes, Chrissy came back and told Rose she needed to go to her boyfriend's car and take him some papers and she was off after Rose said, "Obviously nobody wants to know about Film Ops [their booth's company name], we're not busy, I'll hold down the fort."

I was thinking that it was going *way* too smoothly with Rose. Looking back, I did the right thing but I was uncertain at the time. I looked at Rose and said right as she was leaning in towards me feeling comfortable with me and me feeling extremely comfortable with her, and I said, "Well, listen I need to get back to my friends." Her expression took a dive. I took a chance by short-cutting the usual Game time and said, "Here [handing her my phone], Rose put your number in my phone."

She snatched the phone away and did so. She didn't even ask how to enter the number as most do. It turned out she had an Android phone too and knew how to put new names and numbers in the directory. I'm shocked at how much most girls use smart phones but can't put their own numbers in a phone without help.

She then held the phone to her chest and said, "I won't give this back to you until you promise me you'll call me before the day is over!"

I said, "I don't make those kinds of promises Rose!" Then I smiled. Big. Her first – and only – shit test of the day fails to work on me.

Warning: I can tell you from my experience with Rose that when you go 18+ years being a loser and all of a sudden you have this most exquisite girl who wants you and is showing IOIs like crazy, the last thing you will want to do is keep your Alpha Male persona. Being nonchalant with my non-answer to her demand that I call her that very day went against every fiber of my being! But I am as certain as I am writing these words that my ignoring her shit test was what put me over the top with her.

Tip: I have also had this high-speed Game work in a similar manner a few times since Comic-Con. I think the reason I was able to fast-forward the Game a few times is because so many men are so bad at the whole thing. When someone comes along who peacocks, is confident, and who pushes all a woman's buttons properly, she senses she's found someone unusual and begins showing IOIs far faster than non-10s would do.

After I very politely refused her shit test and didn't promise to call her "before the day is over" she said, "At 5:00 today, Chrissy and I are supposed to meet with our Supervisor and the workers at our company's large display booth in Building C. Will you call me at 5:15 because we all have comped dinners at the Marriott Marquee's steak house each night we work. I want you to be my guest there."

I was at a loss. I knew not to accept outright but I was not a fool. This girl for some reason had already made up her mind about me. She was trying to bounce *me* to a new location! But in spite of what it seemed, I assure you that the year before she would not remember me five seconds after I stopped at her booth. I still think it's funny that I was there talking to her and looking at her booth and I never could figure out what her booth was supposed to promote and I still have *no* idea what her company did. Not that I (or anyone else) cared. And I certainly knew not to show enough interest to ask her something so mundane as a question about her company.

I thought quickly and said what I describe next. After only a few months of solid Game practice in the field back home, I had already developed a sixth sense about how to gauge female reactions and how to react to them. I knew not to directly say "Yes" to her dinner invite but I also somehow knew I'd propelled past several stages of typical Game.

I said, "Rose, it's still early in the day. How about this; so far that's certainly the best offer I've had this morning! If none better come along, I'll call at 5:15. If you don't answer, I'll just assume your meeting went longer and maybe it'll work out some other time."

She said, "It will work, just call." I left saying, "If I get a chance, I'll stop by after lunch" and she perked up and smiled at that. With that reaction, I knew not to stop by after lunch. With 10's, absence makes the heart grow fonder.

It's 5:15

All day I saw very little of Comic-Con and saw lots of images of Rose going through my head. That was stupid. There was absolutely no reason it would necessarily work out with her, even the dinner. She might easily change her mind and flake and not answer her cell when I called.

Plus, you should know that the *worst* date early in Game is a dinner date because the conversation can't help but veer off into mediocre talk after a while and it's vital to keep friendly, chatty energy going early in Game. The only date worse is a movie date where you are not the center of her universe.

The one difference here is that if the dinner worked out, it was at a nice place *and* she was getting the check. Well, her company was but the important thing is that I was *not* paying. The more a girl can do for you early in Game, the more she will do for you later. Compliance early is a fantastic sign and one of the best IOIs you can get. One reason for routines such as palm reading is the small compliance test, "Give me your hand" that you use to build into larger compliance tests through the kiss close, bounce, or number close.

I thought 5:15 would never arrive. And that is amazing. It was at the most astounding Comic-Con ever, with stars and authors and companies I cherished all around me and I was only thinking about the possibility with Rose all day.

I should have been keeping up Game! I probably saw 50 more 9's and 10's but paid no attention to them. *That was stupid.* I was putting too much faith in dinner with Rose. You should never do what I did; keep your options open.

Fortunately, things worked out.

At 5:15, I waited seven more minutes. *Never call on* time, especially if she is the one who tells you what time to call. As hard as it was for me to delay, I know it was harder for her to wait.

Tip: If you successfully number close, which you'll do regularly now, and then call her and make a date for coffee or drink another day, *always be late.* If she says anything about your tardiness, say, "You really missed me didn't you?" Don't ever acknowledge her comment directly. Take it almost as though she was describing one of your good points. One advantage is she almost always has purchased a drink by the time you get there so you don't have to buy her one before she's proved herself worthy of it.

Note: Once you've gone out with a girl a time or two, certainly the boyfriend/girlfriend dynamic begins to change things. And when you sleep with her, that sort of changes the relationship too! All the rules of early Game about never calling on time, never being on time for a first date, etc., certainly need modifying as things progress and you get closer to being a "couple." Alphas take care of their female's needs. But only after they take care of yours. In this case, once they show you they care, once they are happy to see you every time you walk into the room, once they have ravished you with kisses a few times before you have a chance to take a breath, well obviously you are going to reciprocate more and more. You move from Game to relationship. You do risk losing some of your Alpha Maleness once you start getting regular sex though. I cannot advise you too strongly to get this for your arsenal *before* that begins to happen: *How to get Almost Instant Obedience from Your Woman.* That book, written by a guy who's named Radu Belasco (is that his real name?) will help ensure that you walk the tightrope between relationship and Alpha Maleness and keeps you with the upper hand even as you begin to show her more respect and possibly eventually love.

At 5:22 I called Rose. She answered on the first ring. Obviously, somebody forgot her "Manual for How 10s Treat Men" book!

She said, "I'm so glad you called! Where are you, I want to see you!" Before I had a chance to answer, she said, "Hey, meet me at my booth from this morning. It's closed but I'll be there in 10 minutes, I just have to get some packets they want us to have for tomorrow and I'll be right there."

So in 15 minutes I was at her booth, and (of course) she was already there. The crowds had thinned out some with the lesser booths closing down and attendees getting something to eat before the nighttime forums and break-out sessions that begin in the evenings.

She beamed when she saw me and said, "David, your caller ID said your last name is Banner, is that right?" I said my phone has magical properties and that it had correctly guessed my last name. I was expecting a Bruce or David Banner joke but none came. She said, "Did you know you're the only guy under 60 I've seen today dressed in a suit?"

A rule of thumb is this: If you don't know a good answer to a girl's question, just wait and let her keep talking. I was unsure if this was going to be a shit test, compliment, or a simple statement of fact. So I waited.

She said, "So I am going to call you Mr. Banner since you're so nicely dressed!"

I said, "I've been called worse" and smiled. I always smile."

She then kiss closed me!

She said, "Your tie there," and she reached for my tie, then she grabbed it and sort of pulled me into her and looked up at me and closed her eyes and kissed me. Right there at the side of her booth. And I'd been doing kiss closes successfully with 9s and 10s for a few months but this did shock my shorts. And it was wonderful. The best kiss I'd ever had. I was Alpha Male but I certainly wasn't going to pull away from that real soon.

We kissed perhaps four minutes and I stopped it (I didn't want to) and I looked at her as I touched her cheek (that touch is always important) and said, "That was quite a surprise. Do you often kiss strangers at Comic-Con?" And she said, "You're not a stranger. I already feel like I know you well and I want to know you better Mr. Banner in a suit."

Then she went back to the spit-swapping.

I stopped it about two minutes later by pulling away a bit, but I kept looking at her. This is *not the time to play hard to get*. I said, "This is wonderful but we're sort of in the line of people still rushing by. Don't we have a dinner to get to? We'll continue this later I assure you."

She said, "Yes, we will Mr. Banner."

She told me that the Hard Rock Hotel (I'd told her and Chrissy earlier where I was staying) was closer than hers and asked if we could we stop there and let her rework her make-up, freshen up a bit, and brush her hair before going to eat and I said certainly. In my mind I was *so thankful I'd gotten the suite and made sure my things were neatly stowed before leaving that morning!*

I figured it's like another bounce, going to my room shows more commitment to me, it builds more trust when I don't attack her there, and she would see I was a guy who had even more DHV because I wouldn't settle for a regular room. So off we went, but not before I did the typical stick-my-arm-out-elbow-toward-her and said, "Take my arm, let's go." She did and we did.

The Dinner

I would like to tell you that we had a delicious dinner, comped by her company, some expensive wine, and a romantic evening walking about San Diego, and all that. But we didn't make it to the dinner. I never got my free steak. It turns out she didn't either.

Our walk to my hotel was amazing and I have to say I was feeling an attraction that the newfound Alpha Male hadn't felt since I'd learned Game. But the walk was great, she did all the talking which is the way it should be when things are good. She did ask what I did back home and I told her that I was also in school, back in Arizona, and that I was studying literature and graphic arts which is why Comic-Con's unique forms of art and film intrigued me enough to attend the conference each year. (She didn't have to know "studying literature and graphic arts" meant I read a lot of comic books. I'd perfected that line already a few months earlier as I was practicing Game.)

When we got to my place, she went to the bathroom and closed the door. Three minutes later she came out and got her day bag she had at Comic-Con and began brushing her hair and talking about how boring it was standing in a booth that nobody cared about all day. And if it wasn't for meeting me and for having Chrissy there she would have gone insane.

I was thinking that she was talking not like a typical 10. She was stunning, had a killer body, had beautiful shoulder-length brown hair that somehow sparkled browns and reds and gold colors all at the same time, her cheekbones were high and almost model-like (without the anorexia), her little butt was as much of a 10 as her face and breasts were, and she was just bubbly and giddy when she talked to me the whole time. Most 10s are more reserved. I liked this New Kind of 10.

I now know it was the attraction to me. Why she didn't have a boyfriend is beyond my imagination because I can't fathom that this wonder of women didn't. But I seriously doubt she did. At one point later she talked about one boy she dated for almost a year that ended badly. I showed an extreme lack of interest but I made note that she possibly could *just now* be emotionally getting over that relationship. Perhaps it had been a couple of months or more and until her trip to San Diego for Comic-Con she had been brooding about things and eventually trying to get back emotionally stable again to date once more. And my timing might have been perfect. Oh... and the suit and the suite of course.

While still at the mirror at my sink, she asked me to come over and help her with her collar. I came up to the mirror behind her, she turned around and put her arms around my shoulders, and the rest was history in the making.

We didn't leave the room until the next morning early when she had to get up to work the booth again Friday. The steak dinner was forsaken for an expensive room service meal that was worth every cent *I* paid for. The indescribable IOIs I had those two hours in my suite before ordering room service deserved me paying for the meal.

Our Time Together

I simply won't go into details. In spite of my being so candid about myself in all other ways in my book, I do want to maintain a respect for Rose and not get gritty about the specifics.

Still, I do know the kinds of things you're wondering and I will address those. First, in spite of being told a *lot* of lies about relationships in our lives, I had heard several times that when it's your first time you will do just fine. Our instincts are all that is needed to handle things well as long as we don't second-guess everything and ruin the moment by talking too much and being too unsure of ourselves.

It was my Game training that kept me from talking too much and certainly I didn't tell her she was my first. (She didn't tell me I was hers either so we were even.) (I wasn't her first obviously.) But that line isn't a lie. You will naturally just do the right things it seems. Just don't over-think it. Game trains you not to over-think such things so when it happens to you, you'll be fine.

Second, that event *is* better than you can imagine it is.

Third, yes she spent the next night with me too. I never got my free steak dinner.

What Now for David and Rose?

She was only working Comic-Con Thursday and Friday. She had to fly back home to Indianapolis Saturday morning about 11:00. I went with her to the airport in her company's rented towncar. I must say, for a company that had a nothing booth at Comic-Con, they sure seemed to throw money around. I think their other booth, the one Rose was at when I called her at 5:22 the first afternoon, that must have been a more retail-oriented booth. At some point she said they were displaying all their products there and it was a large booth staffed by 8 people. I never saw it, or if I did pass it I didn't think anything of it.

The ride to the airport would have been sad I suppose but she was making out with me during most of it. Seriously, we hardly talked that morning so there wasn't much time to get sad at her leaving which I had been sort of worried about. I could *not* show sadness but we did have a great time together, more than I ever thought possible for me at Comic-Con in spite of the fact that I *sort* of planned to get laid there originally. It was more like having a full-time girlfriend than a 2-night stand. And I grew up a lot in just those two days.

I felt ten years older after it was all over because of the experience. Even as she was leaving me to go through security, we kissed a lot, but she was also telling me she needed "exactly you Mr. Banner" at Comic-Con and that it was just what she wanted. She didn't seem sad to be leaving me and I – for some unknown reason even to me now – I wasn't sad either. I was grateful and pleased.

The previous year, if some miracle had happened and I'd even gotten one short kiss from a 6 or a 7, I would have been *in love* and would have probably tried to move to where she lived the moment Comic-Con ended. In the months that passed after Comic-Con, Rose and I have talked a total of four times on the phone. Twice I called her and twice she called me. The conversations were a little strange given what happened there. I think we both realized she's in Indy, I'm in Arizona, and in spite of the gigantic attraction we each had, it sort of was left in San Diego.

We've discussed the possibility of seeing each other but we don't discuss it in detail. We've mentioned how wonderful it would be to "do" Comic-Con again but she is thinking of quitting her job and spending more time at school. She might be seeing someone else. I certainly am. I'm seeing several someone else's.

That's the thing. I have Game to thank for the way Rose and I ended. We ended not sadly, and not with me begging her to like me as the forsaken little twerp I was probably would have done a year earlier. Game was the reason I landed Rose and had such a wonderful time with her. Game was the reason I got laid at Comic-Con with a 10. And Game puts me in the driver's seat for things just like that to happen again.

In the meantime, I am honing my skills and not pining for Rose. Rose is almost certainly gone and unless she calls me, I doubt our paths cross again. I suppose she could see this book and realize it's about us. If so, it's going to be a little embarrassing for me when she learns what a loser I have been most of my life, but I certainly pondered that high and low before deciding to write this in the first place. Plus, I really don't think Rose will mind. She might even have already suspected she was my first because women *do* seem to have a sort of sixth sense about such things. But even if she did, I know it won't matter to either of us. It's more embarrassing that I had to be *taught* how to be liked by a woman like Rose, but isn't that a good thing as opposed to still being a geeky kid who is afraid to speak to them and never learned?

Yes, I think Rose will not mind this a bit. If anything, she might even appreciate knowing what led to our wonderful two nights.

21
IT'S REALLY ABOUT YOU NOW

So.

Six months from now you can be a master at getting all the 9s and 10s you want. Six months from now, you can have your own Rose to think about. The next Comic-Con might be your first Experience. It's up to you.

Think about it. In six months you will be six months older than you are now. You can put this away and think, "I'll get back to it and really master all that stuff!" and then never do it. In six month from now, you will be six months older and you can either be older, wiser, and have a girlfriend or you can be six months older and still lonely.

It truly is up to you. I've done my job.

You have to go out right away and practice opening sets. As you do, you must study the resources in the order I gave them to you. You don't have to study them first, you need to be going out just opening sets and getting your feet wet at the same time as you master the materials in this book and the other resources.

Men, the following is vital that you understand: Game will not fail you. You may fail yourself if you do not practice Game. You can be a winner or a loser. It's not like you have to muster up much to do anything. You know how to walk around girls now, how to talk, how to touch, when to move, when to touch, when to seclude them, how to kiss them (come on admit it, the kiss close is a brilliant and risk-free way to get kissed), when and how to bounce them, and all that.

Your only job is to practice, both by yourself talking aloud so you get the routines down without having to think about them, then practicing your smiling and skills everywhere you go to all men and women of all sizes and ages because you become Alpha Male when you act Alpha Male everywhere. You speak slowly enough to be understood every time. You project so you are heard because Alpha Males know how a "Huh? What did you just say?" ruins a routine's delivery every time and often ends in getting blown-out of the set. You know to practice at clubs keeping the 3-second rule firmly intact so you don't talk yourself out of it when you see a 3-set with a stunning 10 just waiting to be plucked from the set.

But all the hard stuff you never thought you could do? Like trying to go up and ask a 10 out, like trying to think of things to say, like not knowing when to kiss her, none of that hard stuff is needed.

Game makes it easy. It is we who make things hard.

And I've decided something that might just ruin everything for you, but let me say it anyway. Because I think fellow geeks will understand.

I think I am not going for the sex any time soon again.

I think back to Rose and I, and *yea* I think about the sex a *lot*, but what I liked far more was our time together, having that beautiful face smiling *with me* with eyes looking *at me* and with me and only me being close enough to smell her vanilla fragranced hair.

I want that full time.

Game allows me to get laid, and I'm not saying I have that much willpower, but I want to meet the next Rose and stick with her and see how it goes. I got a job at a large financial company here and it's an amazing job for a little high school graduate squirt like me. (Having an uncle for the VP helped.) But I actually have a career with a salary that a lot of college graduates don't get right away. And I think I want to settle down and find my next Rose for the long-term.

I know women enough *now* to know that Rose was an exception. Our amazing early attraction was an anomaly. I'll have to use Game for a while to meet a lot, kiss a lot, call a lot, and date a lot before I find another Rose *but I will find another*. For me, I know I'll be happy with just one.

You have the tools to get as many as you want. I would ask that you think through what you do want though. For most guys like us, a beautiful woman who wants to be with us the rest of our lives is better than most men ever get. And we now have the tools to get that.

I'm going for it.

You should too.